SIVANANDA
beginner's guide to
yoga

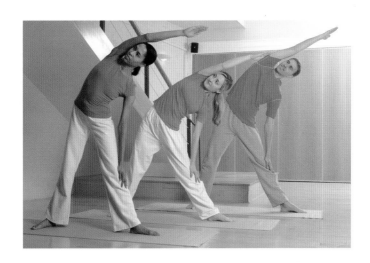

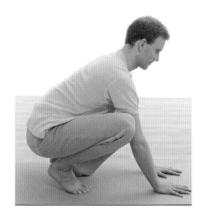
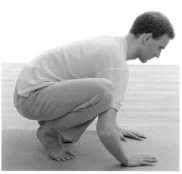
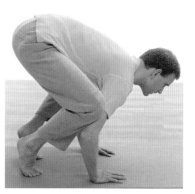

SIVANANDA
beginner's guide to
yoga

The Sivananda Yoga Centre

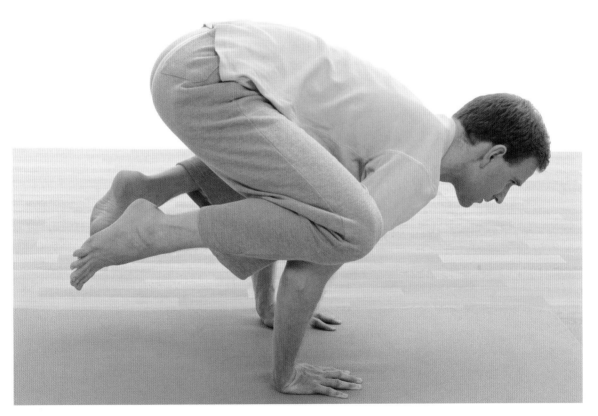

Reconnect with yourself and the planet

Dedicated to Yogiraj Swami Vishnu-devananda

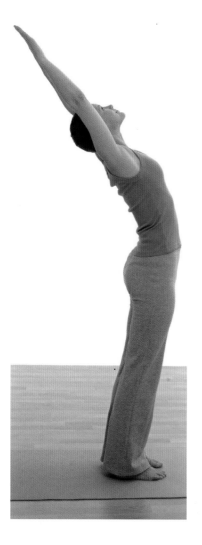

First published in Great Britain in 2006 by
Gaia Books, a division of Octopus Publishing Group Ltd
2–4 Heron Quays, London E14 4JP

Written by Swami Sivadasananda, Yoga Acharya,
sws@sivananda.net

Distributed in the United States and Canada by
Sterling Publishing Co., Inc.
387 Park Avenue South, New York, NY 10016-8810

ISBN-13: 978-1-85675-260-2
ISBN-10: 1-85675-260-7

A CIP catalogue record for this book is available from the
British Library

Printed and bound in China

10 9 8 7 6 5 4 3 2 1

Note

Whilst the advice and information in this book is
believed to be accurate, neither the author nor the
publisher will be responsible for any injury, losses,
damages, actions, proceedings, claims, demands,
expenses and costs (including legal costs or
expenses) incurred or in any way arising out of
following the exercises in this book.

CONTENTS

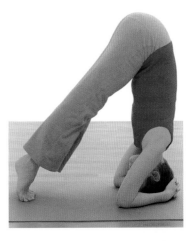

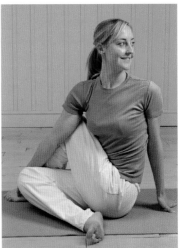

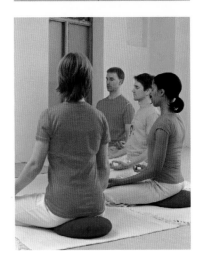

Introduction

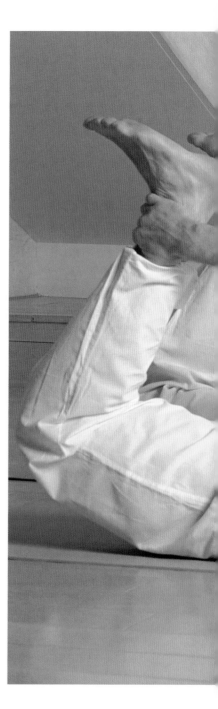

'Yoga balances, harmonizes, purifies and strengthens the body, mind and soul of the practitioner. It shows the way to perfect health, perfect mind control and perfect peace with one's Self, the world, nature and God.'
Swami Vishnu-devananda

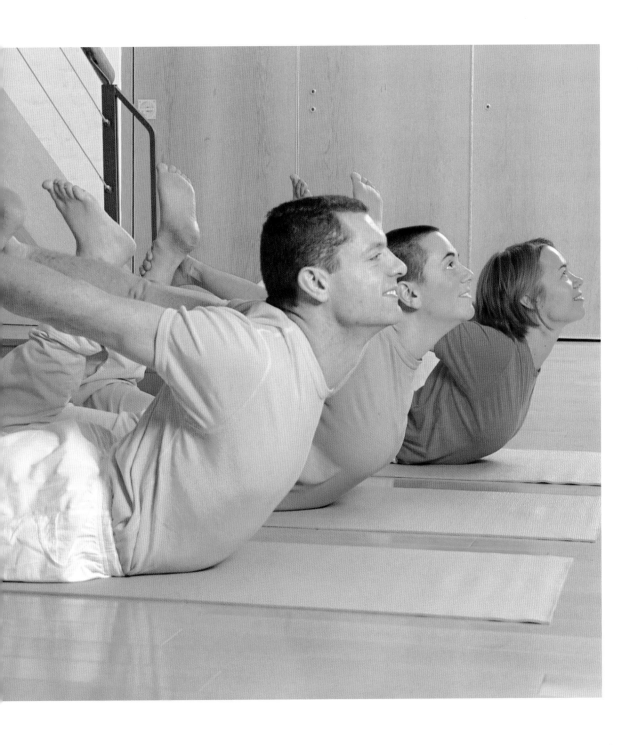

A TIME-HONOURED TRADITION

The divine science of yoga has been practised in India for several thousand years. Based on the search for higher values in life, irrespective of cultural, religious and material background, yoga practice gently tunes both body and mind to the laws of nature.

Yoga is first mentioned in the collection of scriptures called the *Vedas* – the oldest writings found to-date. It is the *Upanishads* – the later part of the *Vedas* – that form the philosophical foundation of yoga teaching. The basic purpose of all yoga is outlined as reuniting the individual self or consciousness (*jiva*) with the Spirit, Supreme Soul or pure consciousness (*Brahman*). Union with this unchanging reality is said to liberate the soul from all sense of separation, freeing it from the illusions of time and space, and allowing us to realize our true nature. In fact, the word *yoga* itself means 'union'. Countless yoga practitioners and teachers the world over have kept this tradition vibrant and alive, reaffirming the classical teachings with their own experience.

Yoga is known as a synthesis of four paths: Jnana Yoga – philosophical inquiry; Bhakti Yoga – devotional practice; Karma Yoga – selfless action; and Hatha or Raja Yoga – body–mind control. Simply put, these paths correspond with a perfect harmony of head (*jnana*), heart (*bhakti*), hands (*karma*) and the inner spirit of humankind (*hatha* or *raja*). This book presents a simple and practical introduction to the path of Hatha, or Raja Yoga.

Great teachers

The preventive and curative effects of yoga are far-reaching and the pioneer work of many yoga

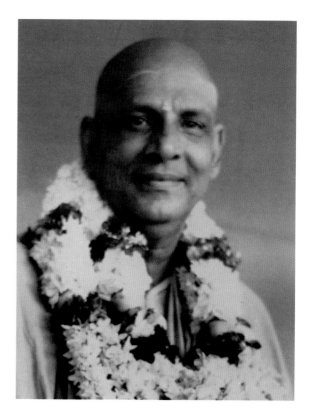

H.H. Swami Sivananda

masters has laid the ground to the broad credibility that yoga enjoys today worldwide.

An inspiring 20th-century embodiment of yoga teachings was H.H. Swami Sivananda (1887–1963). Although he practised and taught yoga in India, his vision was that yoga should benefit the whole world. Having been a doctor before dedicating his life to the path of yoga, H.H. Swami Sivananda presented teachings on yoga in a scientific way, expressing even the most complicated of philosophical subjects in a simple, accessible way. He wrote many authoritative books (mostly in English, which was very uncommon) on all aspects of yoga and established an Ashram, a Yoga Academy. In 1935 he founded an organization known as the Divine Life Society, which is dedicated to the ideals of truth, purity, non-violence, self-realization and world peace. H.H. Swami Sivananda also opened the teachings of yoga to women – a courageous step at a time when India was still under British rule and yoga was taught mainly to men. His foresight is reflected today by the current popularity of yoga, an area in which the majority of practitioners are women.

H.H. Swami Sivananda sent one of his exceptional students, Swami Vishnu-devananda (1927–1993), to the West (initially the United States) in 1957, where he then lived and taught yoga for over 35 years. Swami Vishnu-devananda's dedication and inspired approach to yoga really took hold in North and South America and Europe, as well as in India itself. Under the motto 'clarify and simplify', he taught yoga according to five basic principles (see pages 10–11) in a well-structured sequence of exercises. He also founded the International Sivananda Yoga Vedanta Centres and, after a vision during meditation, started the Yoga Teachers' Training Course as a practical tool for world peace – in line with his great teacher's visions.

Why practise yoga today?

The vast technological progress that has been made in recent decades has resulted in the pace of our lives becoming tremendously fast. Stress relief is therefore the number one reason for the practice of yoga today (see pages 12–15). The simplicity of practising yoga on a small mat on the floor offers an all-too-welcome contrast to the complexity of modern life, gradually allowing the body and mind to regain their balance. While many people are initially drawn to yoga to combat stress, to keep their bodies fit and flexible, or to seek relief from a specific complaint, such as backache, many also end up experiencing subtle changes in their approach to life as they begin to understand the inner peace that is their true nature.

For beginners, the benefits of yoga are mostly felt as mechanical changes in joints and muscles, increased blood circulation, temperature changes and improved control of the nervous system through regulated breathing. According to yogic teachings, all of these are really changes in *prana* currents (shifts in the vital life energy that runs through every life form), which, as practitioners become more rooted and sensitive in the exercises, they will start to experience on a mental level as well as a physical one. Understanding and controlling *prana* – the subtle energy in all life forms – is viewed as the key to healthy body–mind balance.

Swami Vishnu-devananda

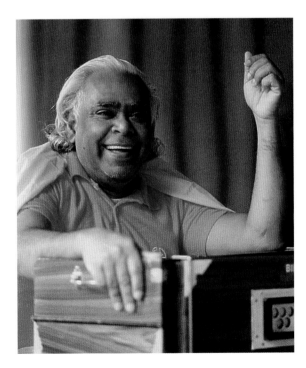

THE FIVE BASIC PRINCIPLES

By closely observing the lifestyles and needs of people in the West, Swami Vishnu-devananda (see page 9) condensed the ancient wisdom of yoga into five basic principles, which he felt could be easily incorporated into Westerners' living patterns to improve their quality of life. The five principles are explained below, and it is around these that this book is based.

Proper exercise

Yoga offers a complete but relatively gentle form of physical exercise, without the potential side effects of muscle fatigue and over-stimulation that tend to be experienced with other fitness programmes. The postures, called asanas in Sanskrit (meaning firm and comfortable pose), can be practised by people of all ages and from

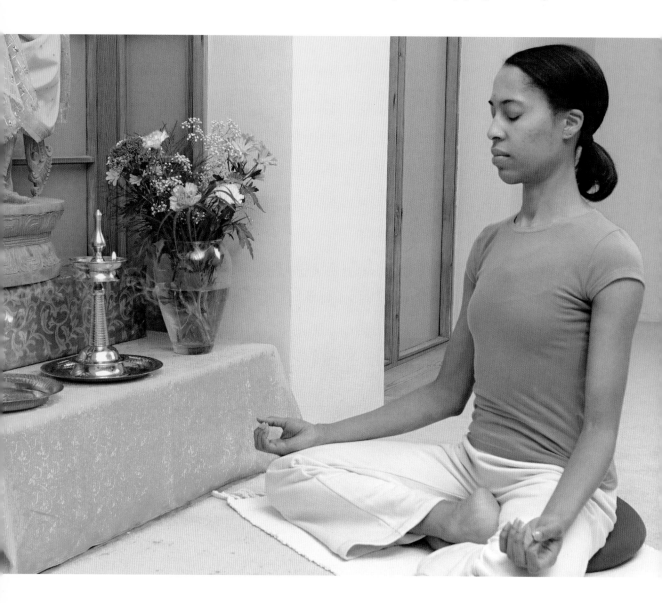

all walks of life at a level that suits their individual needs. The asanas give excellent lubrication to the body's machinery of joints, muscles and ligaments, creating a strong and flexible spine, stretching and toning the body, enhancing the digestive process, improving circulation, increasing *prana* (the vital energy that runs through every life form) and boosting powers of concentration. The muscle-stretching and contraction involved also brings rest and regeneration to all body systems. Chapter 1 offers eight progressive classes of yoga exercises from which you can benefit (see pages 22–127).

Proper breathing

Full, rhythmical breathing makes use of all, not just part, of the lungs to maximize oxygen intake. Physical activity automatically stimulates this type of deep breathing, but often, in modern society, people have non-physical jobs that entail sitting at a desk or computer all day. Unfortunately, this does not encourage full breathing, despite the fact that the brain requires more oxygen for efficient mental work than any other organ or muscle does to function optimally. Yoga breathing techniques are designed to enable you to make full use of your lung capacity and therefore maximize your oxygen intake even when sitting stationary. Improving your breathing habits will lead to increased vitality, and doing a few rounds of breathing exercises each day (see pages 38–41, 60–61 and 86–87 in Chapter 1) will thoroughly 'recharge your batteries'.

Proper relaxation

Relaxation is an important and integral part of yoga, as it gives you a chance to let go of your worries and stresses, it releases tensions from all your muscles and it rests your whole system, leaving you feeling rejuvenated. Yoga relaxation techniques allow you not only to overcome existing stress symptoms, but also to develop a greater resistance to further external stress factors. Relaxation exercises are recommended between all main yoga exercises in Chapter 1 (see pages 46–47) to rest the body before the next exercise, and Final Relaxation (see pages 54–57) acts like a cooling system for both the body and mind.

Proper diet

According to yogic teachings, a fresh, well-balanced vegetarian diet is key to developing and maintaining physical and mental strength (see pages 130–133). The subtle components of each meal provide the nutrients that the organs and muscles need to function optimally. Your age, the climate in which you live, what season it is and the type of work you perform, as well as your body type (see page 135) should be considered when making your food choices. The whole of Chapter 2 (see pages 128–143) guides you in why and how to maintain a 'proper diet'.

Positive thinking and meditation

The mind can be considered as the intelligent driver of your body vehicle. It is therefore important to train it – in the form of positive thinking and meditation – so that it understands the aim of life's journey and how to arrive at your desired destination. Positive thinking (see pages 148–149) develops higher emotions such as courage, love and contentment, which progressively substitute negative impulses such as fear, anger, jealousy or impatience. And the practice of meditation (see pages 152–155) allows the mind to become still, like a lake without waves, leading you towards inner peace – the treasure at the bottom of the lake, which can only be found once all thoughts subside.

OVERCOMING STRESS

Most aspects of the average modern lifestyle are run at great speed. We tend to try to fit more and more into our lives, with heavier workloads, more demands on our time, greater distances to travel to our destinations, and higher expectations. Different people experience stress in different ways, and while stress symptoms can be clearly diagnosed, there is no common medical solution for them. There are, however, many possible ways of trying to deal with feelings of stress – from doing sport, having a massage and taking nerve tonics to going on vacation, changing jobs or trying to develop a more positive outlook on life.

Yoga is also an extremely popular and effective system for bringing about relief from stress, and is complementary to all of the options listed above. So, exactly how does the combination of postures, breathing exercises and relaxation techniques described in Chapter 1's eight classes (see pages 22–127) allow you to 'stretch away your stress'?

The 'fight or flight' response

Feelings of stress are not directly caused by specific external factors; they come about due to the body's instinctive response to these external factors, known as 'fight or flight'. As part of the survival instinct, this is a very useful reaction: it is activated when we are confronted with imminent threats, such as a natural catastrophe or a direct physical attack. At such times, we literally need to face up to a situation ('fight' for our life) or flee from it ('flight') to save our lives.

Time pressure, emotional conflicts, financial worries, pollution, competitive environments and excessive noise cannot be compared with an imminent physical threat, yet our nervous system interprets them in the same way. The activity of certain body systems is put on high alert, while other systems are temporarily slowed down. These changes actually create the strong subjective impression that we are undergoing a life-threatening physical emergency. Depending on the situation, the body starts to behave as though there is really somebody we should fight or from whom we should run away.

Stress symptoms

Part of the autonomic (involuntary) nervous system, sympathetic nerves originate from the thoracic (central) and lumbar (lower) area of the spine, from where they spread out to many of the body's systems, sending news of the apparent 'emergency' at times of stress. As the name suggests, we have no conscious control over this part of the nervous system, so we do not know that these nerves have been activated until we experience actual stress symptoms.

Increased strength and speed of heartbeat: Blood is pumped around the body faster to provide the muscles with the oxygen they supposedly need to respond to the situation. When this reaction sets in, any kind of quiet, concentrated activity (including sleep) becomes very difficult.

Changes in the digestive system: Blood is directed away from the digestive organs to skeletal muscles, basically shutting down the digestive system. This means that any food eaten during this time is likely to sit in the stomach for a long time, putting unnecessary strain on the body.

Increased contraction in the skeletal muscles: Under stress, many major muscles contract in expectation of either fight (mainly the neck and shoulder muscles) or flight (mainly the leg muscles). As well as being uncomfortable, these contractions use up large amounts of vital energy, causing you to feel physically tired at the end of a stressful day, even if very little muscular work has been done.

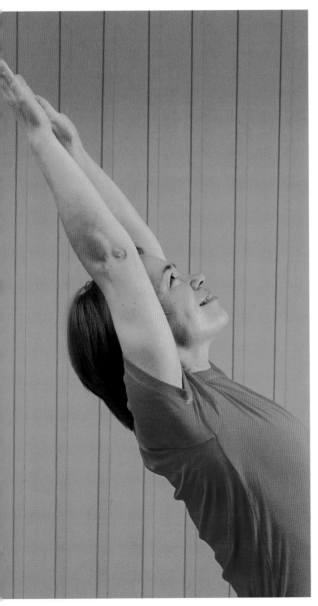

Increased rate of breathing: Under stress, the solar plexus becomes tense and prevents healthy abdominal breathing (see pages 38–41). Instead, you inhale into the chest and exhale only in a short, superficial way. This incapacity to exhale in a relaxed way creates feelings of anxiety and can make it difficult to speak quietly or use long sentences without becoming breathless.

Increased glucose levels: Under stress, glucose levels become higher in the blood, causing the hormone insulin to be released from the pancreas in order to use up the extra blood sugar. This insulin release can be quite strong, resulting in a sudden drop in blood sugar levels, which is why we often feel hungry after a stressful event. If stress becomes habitual, a typical reaction is to crave and eat a lot of sweet food.

Exercise the stress away

Many doctors advise sport as a natural way to 'work out' stress, yet it is interesting to see how many sports actually imitate the 'fight or flight' situation. Most sporting games are either physical or psychological combat situations, which stimulate and express the fighting instinct: 'winning' is the aim. By contrast, different types of running or walking (including running machines) imitate 'flight'.

In the yoga exercise system, Sun Salutation (see pages 64–71) is a gentle and non-competitive way to work out the urge to be active. You can gradually speed up movements, as long as you maintain deep, rhythmical breathing. In this way you don't add new stress, due to tense movements, to your nervous system. When you are lying in Final Relaxation afterwards (see pages 54–57), you can actually feel how the activity of the sympathetic (stress-activating) nervous system already has calmed down.

Rest and repair

The parasympathetic nerves, another part of the autonomic (involuntary) nervous system, originate from below the brain and from the sacral (lower) area of the spine. They connect to exactly the same organs as the sympathetic nerves, but their effect is opposite. They generate 'rest and repair' in the organs, which means that they tell the body to return to normal once the 'emergency scenario' of the stress reaction is over. The parasympathetic message consists of:

- Slowing down the heartbeat
- Slowing down breathing patterns
- Promoting digestive gland secretion
- Encouraging the digestive processes
- Stimulating bowel movement
- Increasing secretion of tears and saliva

Like any other nerves, parasympathetic nerves need to be activated in order to transmit their message. While the sympathetic (stress-activating) nervous system is stimulated automatically, the parasympathetic (calm-inducing) nervous system needs to be activated consciously, other than during deep, relaxed sleep. This is why you may feel incapable of 'just relaxing' in a stressful situation. However, through yoga, you can learn how to do this.

Stretch the stress away

When a newcomer to yoga stretches a muscle during a posture, at a certain point it becomes slightly uncomfortable. During the first classes of the Yoga Programme (see Chapter 1), the stretch is maintained for a short time only and is

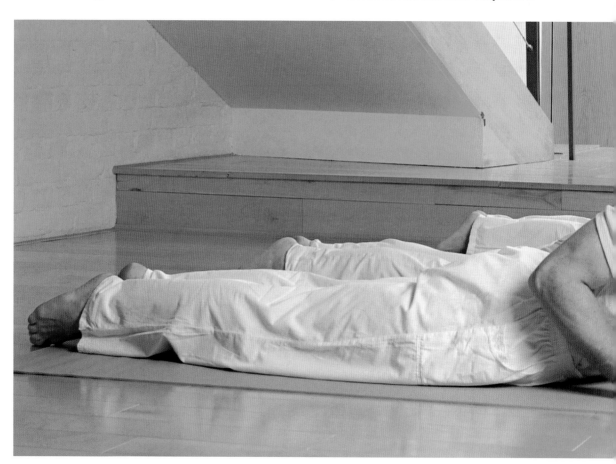

followed immediately by relaxation. This rhythmical alternation of stretch discomfort and relaxation progressively relaxes the tense muscle and activates the parasympathetic reaction, creating a sensation of relaxed well-being. By the time you reach Final Relaxation (see pages 54–57), you can literally feel the process of rest and repair in every cell in your body from your head down to your feet.

Relax the stress away

Towards the second half of the programme, the yoga postures demand more active muscle contractions (rather than just stretching), especially in asanas such as the Cobra (see pages 80–82), the Locust (see pages 90–91) and the Bow (see pages 96–97). These muscle

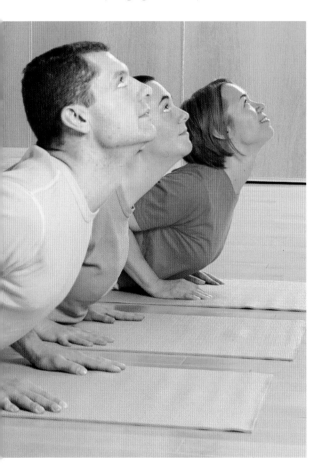

contractions create relaxation on an even deeper level because many hidden tensions are released from the muscle fibres when the muscles relax after a strong contraction. This increased relaxation after a muscular effort prepares the mind to accept the challenges of daily life in a more relaxed way.

Yoga is the key

In summary then, yoga exercises reduce the over-stimulation of the sympathetic nervous system and activate the 'rest and repair' of the parasympathetic nervous system. Daily practice is a guaranteed protection against stress, because the benefits last for up to 24 hours. Stressful living conditions may continue to stimulate the sympathetic nervous system, for example by asking your heartbeat to accelerate or your digestion to slow down, but the activated parasympathetic nervous system effectively counteracts the stimulation, allowing you to remain relaxed. And even if, due to overwhelming circumstances, you experience some stress reactions, you can keep your cool because you know that these symptoms will disappear once you do your yoga session in the evening.

The yoga approach to stress management is first of all to create a stress-free experience each time you practise yoga, so be sure to find a quiet, clean, clutter-free space in which you will remain uninterrupted for the duration of each yoga class. It is also important, through self-observation, to develop your awareness of any physical or mental habits that may be allowing unnecessary stress, whether unhealthy eating, negative thinking or simply not allowing any 'down time' for yourself. Yoga advocates practical lifestyle tips, ranging from a healthy vegetarian diet to positive thinking and meditation exercises, which will help to eliminate such self-created stress conditions.

CONSERVING VITAL ENERGY

Yoga teaches that the same *prana*, or vital life
energy, vibrates in different wavelengths in
body movements, involuntary functions such as
digestion, activity of the mind and sensory
activity. What is measured in athletic sports
competitions is the amount of *prana* that can be
projected into the physical effort. In a car-racing
competition, the best driver is he who excels in
coordinating the *prana* with precision both in the
physical effort and the sensory perception. In a
chess competition, the same projection of *prana*
occurs during strategic thinking.

What is common in all these situations is that
the *prana* is measured at the very moment it is
actually being spent. Similarly, when we enjoy
basic activities such as eating, talking, shaking
hands or listening to music, we unconsciously
stimulate an outflow of *prana*.

During the practice of yoga postures,
breathing techniques and relaxation, on the other
hand, only a minimum amount of *prana* is used
and a lot is conserved, which can then be used at
will in daily life for all types of activities.

The yogic way to balance the accumulation
and spending of *prana* is related to a finely tuned
use of the five senses: touching, seeing, hearing,
tasting and smelling. Yoga provides training that
allows greater precision in sensory perception on
one hand, while on the other, it enables the
senses to withdraw from disturbing sensory input
on the other.

When you closely observe the functioning of
the five senses, you can discover new ways to
experience them in a more balanced way. This is
in great contrast to the usual daily bombardment
and over-stimulation of our senses, which
requires the use of lots of *prana*.

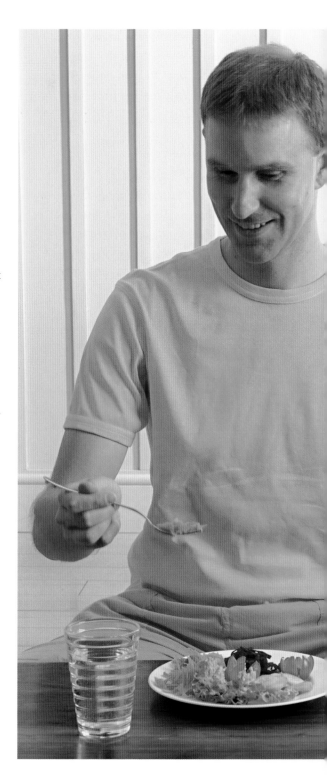

Touch

The skin or sense of touch includes the sense of pressure, temperature and pain, and is associated with millions of sensory receptors in the skin, internal organs and muscles. As such, it relates to body awareness in general.

When practising an asana or posture, sensations of pressure, temperature and, occasionally, discomfort are increased, activating the sense of touch. In order to feel and identify all these sensory impressions, *prana* is projected towards the body. Once you relax, the sensations of pressure, temperature and pain return to a harmonious sensation of well-being as the *prana* is conserved. This sense of 'subtle touch' heightens your sense of touch when it comes to external objects and people.

Sight

Many yoga exercises improve the vitality and proper functioning of the eyes. For example, *tratak*, or steady gazing, (see page 154) cleanses the eyes by stimulating tears; Eye Exercises (see pages 31–33) relax and strengthen the eye muscles; and inverted poses, such as Shoulderstand (see pages 50–53) and Headstand (see pages 126–127), increase circulation in the eyes. Simply lying down on your back and closing your eyes in Corpse Pose (see pages 28–29) will give great relief to strained eyes. However, a deeper rest for the physical sense of sight comes with a relaxed contemplation of a mental image (see page 154) as this relates to the inner capacity of seeing.

Hearing

Yoga practice expands hearing. The classes in Chapter 1 include repeating the universal sound OM (see pages 30 and 57: OM Chanting and Final Relaxation). The difference in sound perception at the beginning and at the end of the class is astonishing. When singing OM after Final Relaxation, the sound is actually perceived in the whole body as a subtle vibration.

As well as governing the sense of hearing, the inner ear also controls the sense of balance. The practice of balancing poses, such as the Crow, (see pages 114–115), the Tree (see page 116) and the Peacock (see page 117), in yoga can help to increase your sense of balance and general body awareness.

Taste

When you follow yogic recommendations and opt for a vegetarian diet, the fresh, organic foods mildly spiced with fresh herbs offer a whole new range of taste sensations, which will make you more sensitive to subtle flavours. It is believed that over-spiced food is too heavy to digest (using up a lot of *prana*), whereas mildly spiced food is lighter and easier to digest, allowing you to conserve *prana*. Once you get used to the more subtle tastes of a vegetarian diet, you will have a double advantage: feeling satisfied and conserving *prana*.

Sense of smell

Yogic cleansing exercises, called *kriyas*, such as *jala neti* (see pages 138–139), remove excess mucus from the nasal cavity, improving your sense of smell.

Yogic understanding is that the olfactory nerve is an extension of what can be called the 'emotional brain', and therefore a direct link between the brain and physical breathing. The science of *pranayama* (breath regulation; see pages 86–89) offers techniques that not only increase the absorption of *prana* in the body, but also directly balance the emotions and help to improve concentration.

LEARNING TO RELAX

Deep relaxation requires you to understand and try to change certain ways in which you habitually think and act. The body in itself is always ready to relax, as this would allow it to function in the most efficient way, but it needs to receive the adequate relaxation command from the mind. This can be compared to a car, which is ready to go absolutely anywhere, but needs to be driven by a driver who knows the basic functioning of the car and the most suitable route to reach the destination.

In yoga, the word detachment is often used to describe the capacity needed in order to relax and 'let go' of habitual thoughts, worries and stresses in the mind. As well as learning physical relaxation techniques to help to promote this, it is important to gain a basic understanding of how relaxation works on a mental level.

The conscious and subconscious mind

The subconscious mind not only controls the autonomic nervous system, but also contains the functions of memory, instincts and emotions. The term 'subconscious' suggests that we do not have awareness of or control over these functions. However, there are, in fact, many ways to influence the subconscious mind.

Childhood education leaves deep impressions in the subconscious mind and programmes basic values and principles. Habitual activities are another aspect of the subconscious mind: many daily activities such as walking, eating or driving a car tend to be done in a habitual, non-thinking manner. This includes the possibility of negative programming in the case of addictions, for example.

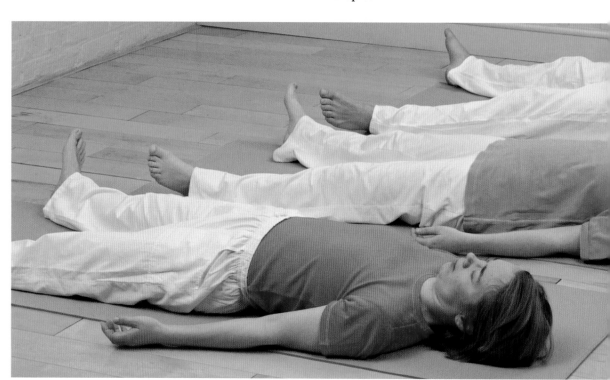

Self-observation, attention, willpower, clear understanding, thorough reasoning and abstract thinking are all, on the other hand, functions of the conscious mind. What is commonly called the power of personality is related to the development of the conscious mind. Psychology uses the intellect to understand the nature of the mind, and philosophy applies reasoning to understand the relationship between ourselves and the Universe.

In order to develop the capacity for deep relaxation, yoga suggests that you try to become aware (via your conscious mind) of subconsious patterns of behaviour that may be preventing you from completely relaxing or from leading a healthy lifestyle – whether these are things that have been ingrained from childhood or habits that have developed over time. During relaxation of the internal organs (see page 55) it is actually the subconscious mind that delivers the relaxation message.

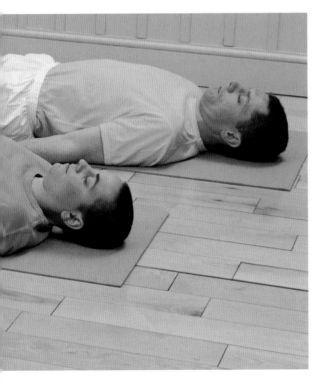

Non-attachment: the key to relaxation

Most people think of attraction or liking as a positive element in life, but, in yogic terms, when associated with objects of the material world, this attitude brings tension, which makes complete relaxation very difficult. This is because 'liking' leads to desires, which can in turn lead to a sense of frustration if these desires are not met (see page 20).

Attraction also brings with it a constant fear of loss. After all, nothing is permanent in the physical world, which means that loss cannot be avoided. Aversion or dislike brings pain, too: it is a negative attitude that often makes a neutral situation appear as if it were one to be avoided. Learning to be content in all circumstances is the key to relaxation.

It is therefore useful to try to phase out overly emotional reactions to individuals and situations. A good first step is to observe the way you often talk in daily life. 'I like that', 'This is lovely', 'This is great', 'I hate that', 'I don't like that' and 'This is terrible', are common expressions of like and dislike, which you probably use quite often. If you try to start using such expressions less often, you will become less 'attached' to whatever is going on around you. This non-attachment should not be confused with a generally passive attitude and certainly does not mean that you should feel less love and compassion; it simply means that you can observe emotions in a slightly distanced fashion as they arise and can then put them aside.

Non-attachment is a state of mind. It is not running away from society, duties and responsibilities. It simply involves being unattached to the pulls of likes and dislikes, bringing about a sense of inner contentment and, with it, an ability to completely relax.

PRACTICAL YOGA PHILOSOPHY

The following definitions present the main aspects of practical yoga philosophy and have been extracted from the works of the great Yoga Master, H.H. Swami Sivananda. They propose affirmative ideals that will greatly enrich and enhance your experience of yoga.

The Self

The Self, or Supreme Soul, is the essential nature of man – the common consciousness in all beings. A thief, a prostitute, a king, a saint, a dog, a cat, a rat – all are in essence the same common Self. Full awareness of the Self, which can be attained through yoga, is bliss itself.

Ignorance

It is due to ignorance that we perceive diversity rather than unity. The apparent difference between the individual, the world and the Self is only an illusion. This illusion works at great speed through the fluctuations and imaginations of the mind. However real time and space may appear, they are mental creations, as unreal as dreams. The timeless, spaceless Self is the only reality.

Liberation

By breaking down the barriers of separate existence, the unity of the Self can be experienced. It is not attainment of liberation from an actual state of bondage, but it is the realization of the liberation that already exists. It is freedom from a false notion of bondage.

Desire

The cause of ignorance or the 'apparent bondage' mentioned above is desire. Desire creates thoughts that veil the real nature of the Soul, which is blissful and eternal. Practically speaking, there is nothing wrong with having desires and satisfying them. The problem is that no matter how many you satisfy, new ones constantly arise, creating endless frustration. When desires are, on the other hand, reduced and finally transcended through self-discipline, intuitive knowledge of the Self dawns on the individual.

Reason

Intellect and reason are finite instruments that can achieve wonders in the realm of finite duality,

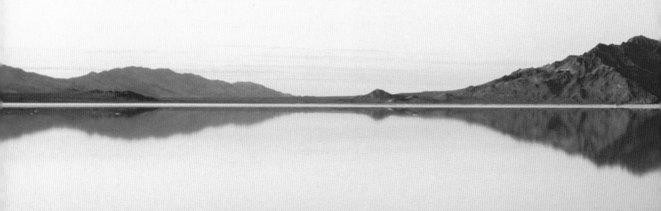

but are powerless in the realm of infinite non-duality. For example, reason or logic can design and build a space shuttle (duality), but it can not give a satisfying answer to the question 'Who am I?' (non-duality). Knowledge of the Self is a non-dual, intuitive experience; while the dualistic knowledge of objects through mind and senses, is a mere knowledge of appearance.

Intuition

Intuition dawns like a flash. It does not grow bit by bit. The immediate knowledge of intuition unites the individual soul with the Self, or Supreme Soul. Intuitive knowledge is imperishable knowledge of the Truth. Without developing intuition, the intellectual man remains imperfect. Meditation leads to intuition.

Matter and spirit

The fundamental error of all ages is the belief that the spiritual and material worlds are separate. Matter is really Spirit seen through the senses. The world is an expression of the Self or the Absolute. Matter is the Power of the Supreme Soul. It is the light that shines in various forms, the one voice that speaks in various languages, the one life that thrills through every atom in the universe.

Good and evil

All life is alike. Just as one thread penetrates all flowers in a garland, so also one Self penetrates all living beings. The world is neither good nor bad. The mind creates good and evil. To a good person, the world is full of good, but to the bad, the world is full of evil. The evil is not in the world; it is in the mind. By seeing the Self everywhere, good can be seen everywhere.

Unity of existence

There is only one race, the race of humanity. None is high, none is low, all are equal. Man-made barriers should be ruthlessly broken down. Humanity is one single family.

Yoga and religion

Religion is a manifestation of the eternal glow of the Spirit within man. The main purpose of religion is the unfoldment of divinity within man. Religion is living, not speaking or showing. Real religion is religion of the heart.

CHAPTER 1

The Yoga Programme

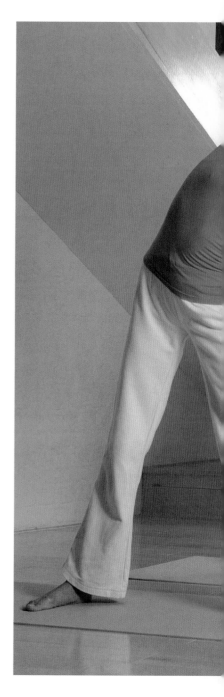

'Yoga is not a matter of erudition; its roots lie in action. It must be lived to be learned. It is in oneself, and not others, that the rich source of inner development must be sought. Growth comes, but is gradual. Sincerity, regularity and patience will ensure eventual advancement.'

Swami Vishnu-devananda

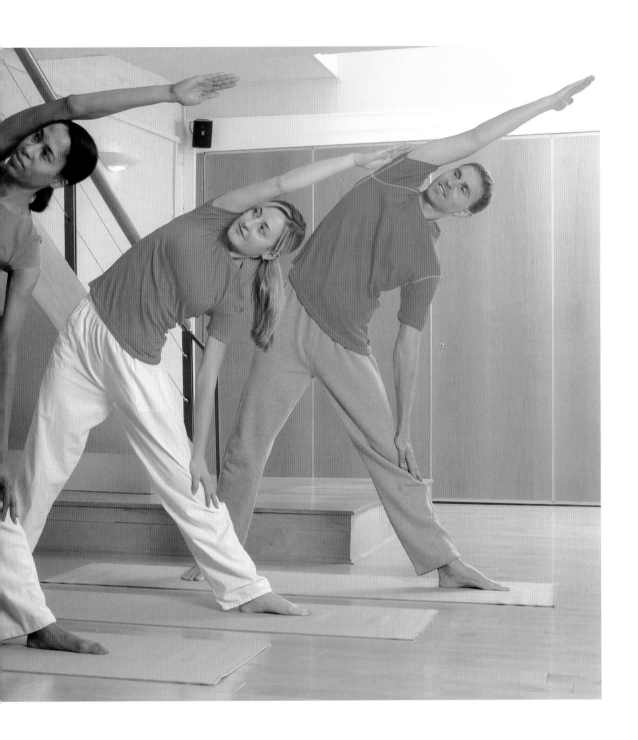

HOW THE PROGRAMME WORKS

The gentle yoga programme in the following pages is divided into eight progressive classes, each of which provides a balanced yoga session that will leave you feeling relaxed and full of energy. The classes cover three of the five basic principles of yoga: Proper Exercise, Proper Breathing and Proper Relaxation, while Proper Diet and Positive Thinking and Meditation are dealt with in Chapters 2 and 3 (see pages 128–143 and 144–155).

Natural progression

Each class is a progression of the previous one, culminating in Class 8, which includes all 12 basic asanas: Headstand, Shoulderstand, the Plough, the Fish, Forward Bend, the Cobra, the Locust, the Bow, Half Spinal Twist, the Peacock (or the Crow), Standing Forward Bend and the Triangle.

At the start of each class, an exercise plan outlines the contents of that session, leading you back to previous chapters for guidance on certain exercises and postures, and leading you forward for explanations of new ones. Make sure that you include the relaxation poses indicated between exercises, as these are integral to a complete yoga practice.

It is best to do any one class at least three times before moving onto the next level but, after this, just be guided by your own experience about what feels comfortable for you. If you do not feel confident about trying some of the new exercises in a certain class, it is fine to choose just a few of them, while continuing to do the exercises that you already know from the previous class. Be sure, however, that you sit calmly and read through the whole class that you intend to do, before actually starting to do it.

As well as the detailed instructions for the actual practice, you will find a variety of additional information such as the benefits of each exercise and preparations that guide you in a step-by-step way for a full posture if needed. There are also 'adaptations' that offer a different approach for people experiencing limitations, and 'variations' that show the same exercise from a slightly different angle to allow a more complete experience. Just use these in whatever way is most useful for you.

Importance of regularity

Although it will be the physical experience of the exercises and postures that affects you most strongly at first, you will grow more aware of the flow of *prana*, or vital energy, and of the importance of deep breathing and relaxation as you progress. Do not be discouraged if your progress seems slow at first and your postures, or asanas, seem to bear little resemblance to those illustrated. Regular practice will steadily narrow the gap, as will a positive approach. Above all, never force or strain yourself to get into a posture. You will only ever improve when your muscles are relaxed.

Setting the scene

Never practise yoga on a full stomach; it is best to do it between two and three hours after a meal, and aim to have a meal or a snack soon after you have completed the session. Wear fresh, loosely fitting cotton clothes that will not restrict your breathing or movement; take off any jewellery to reduce restrictions on the skin; and remove glasses or hard contact lenses. Choose a practice space that is clean, clutter-free and well-ventilated and try to do your yoga at a time when you are likely to remain undisturbed throughout the session. It is best to practise on a mat of some sort – either a folded blanket or a rubber exercise mat.

How much time is needed?

A general time frame is given for each class at the start of its own section in the book. The exercise instructions themselves then give an indication of how many times a movement should be repeated or how long a pose should be held for. Besides that, it is best not to worry too much about time. If, for some reason, a class takes you much longer than you expected and you need to finish before completing the class, you may do so at any time. Just make sure you do the complete final relaxation with autosuggestion before leaving the exercise mat (see pages 54–56).

You may find that you do not always have enough time to do a full class. In this instance, you can do a shorter practice by following the circle symbol or triangle symbol. These split each class, other than Class 1, which needs to be done in its entirety, into two separate sessions, each of which provides a well-rounded yoga session. Remember that doing a little regularly is better than doing a lot occasionally, so try to do your practice either every day or every other day.

Special precautions

If you suffer from any serious disease or have a spinal injury, see your doctor before you take up yoga practice. Women should avoid inverted postures during menstruation.

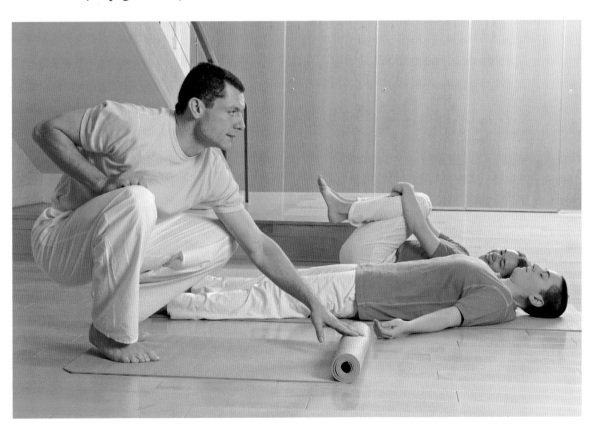

Class 1

This first class consists of a few simple stretches and just one asana – Shoulderstand – forming a gentle introduction to yoga bodywork. It also covers two other important aspects of yoga: how to breathe properly and how to relax. As you read the explanations in detail, you will gradually become aware of the precision and sound physiological basis of all yoga exercises.

Becoming familiar with Class 1 before progressing onto the others is somewhat like learning the alphabet before being able to write single words, form sentences and tell a complete story. Just as you have to refer back to single letters and single words when writing a story, you will have to refer back to the basic yoga building blocks of this class at times when you start doing the later classes.

Although very simple in appearance, this class introduces you to all the main tools for your future yoga practice – a combination of postures, breathing and relaxation. It is therefore vital that you practise it at least three times in its entirety before moving on to Class 2. As H.H. Swami Sivananda wisely said: 'An ounce of practice is better than a ton of theory.'

How long does the class take?
30 minutes to read through the class
45–60 minutes to practise it for the first time
30–45 minutes to repeat the practice

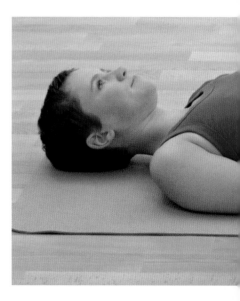

EXERCISE PLAN

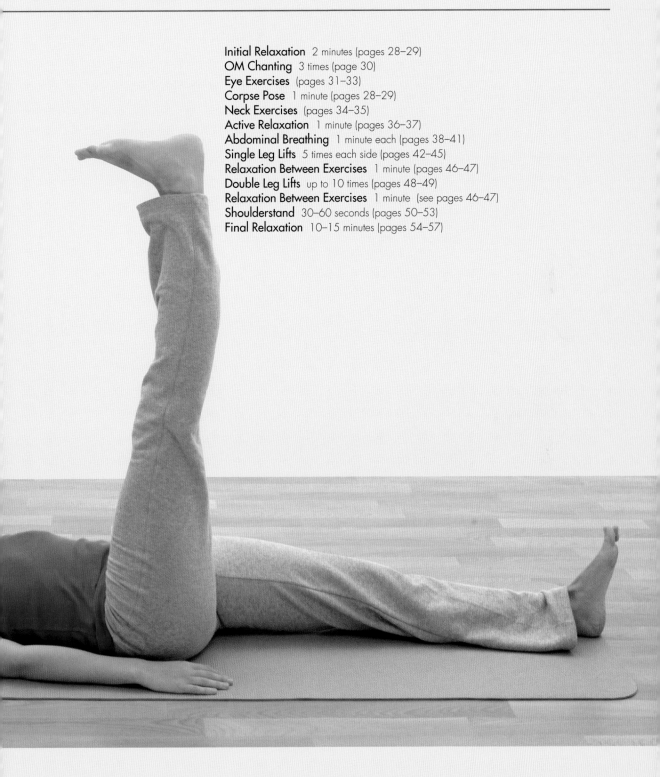

INITIAL RELAXATION

Savasana

Relaxing on your back in what is known as Corpse Pose helps the body to absorb correct alignment. At first glance, it looks as though you are doing nothing. However, as you discover the various relaxation practices throughout the yoga programme, you will develop a whole new awareness of your body and its natural capacity to rest and balance itself. If it feels uncomfortable going straight into Corpse Pose for any reason, you could do one of the variations provided - just choose whichever one seems most suitable for your needs.

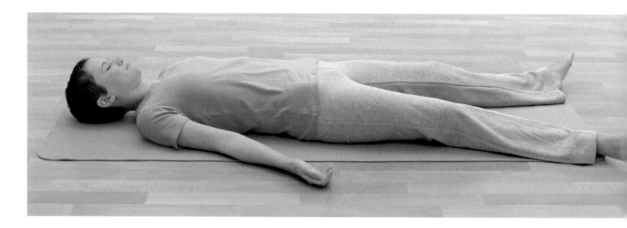

Corpse Pose

Lie comfortably on your back, with your legs and arms apart, your feet released to the side and your palms facing upwards. Make sure that you release the weight of your lower back towards the floor, close your eyes and breathe in and out slowly and rhythmically through your nose. As you inhale, let your abdomen expand and as you exhale, let it come down again. Feel your body becoming heavy and relaxed with each exhalation. Do this for up to 2 minutes.

Corpse Pose Variations

If Corpse Pose causes any problems or discomfort in your lower
back, you may want to do one of the following variations before
going into or while in the full posture. With time, the yoga exercises
in the rest of this class will start to improve your spinal alignment
and flexibility, allowing you to go straight into Corpse Pose.

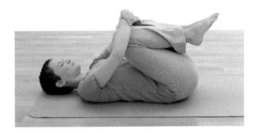

VARIATION 1

*Lie on your back, bend your legs in
towards your chest and hug your arms
around your knees, holding one wrist
with the opposite hand. Take 5 deep
breaths, allowing your lower back to
gently stretch and relax against the
floor. Then release your legs into full
Corpse Pose.*

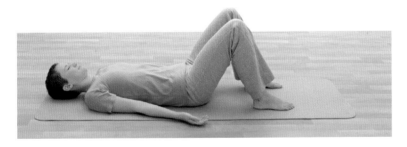

VARIATION 2

*Lie on your back, bend your legs and
place your feet flat on the floor, keeping
your legs apart. Take 5 deep breaths,
allowing your lower back to relax
against the floor. Then release your legs
into full Corpse Pose.*

VARIATION 3

*To reduce any exaggerated curvature
of the lower back and provide comfort
for this area, place a pillow or rolled-
up towel under each knee while
in Corpse Pose.*

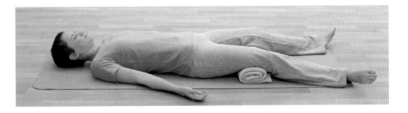

VARIATION 4

*If your upper spine has an
exaggerated curvature (kyphosis)
and you experience discomfort when
releasing your head to the floor in
Corpse Pose, place a small folded
towel under your head.*

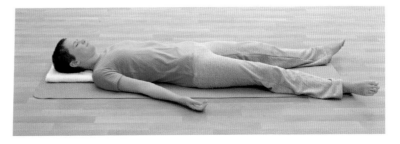

OM CHANTING

OM chanting provides increased body–mind harmony, which is necessary for a successful yoga session, not only helping you to focus on doing the exercises, but also making you more body- and mind-aware while doing them. Some of the meditation techniques that are explained in detail on pages 154–155 are applied here in miniature to calm the mind.

OM is considered to be the universal sound of creation, out of which all the letters of the Sanskrit alphabet evolved. It consists of three sounds A, U and M, which cover the full range of sounds possible for the human voice. The sound vibration when chanting it starts in the navel with the sound O and is taken up slowly to the sound M vibrating in the 'third eye chakra' (see page 153), expanding further to the top of the head.

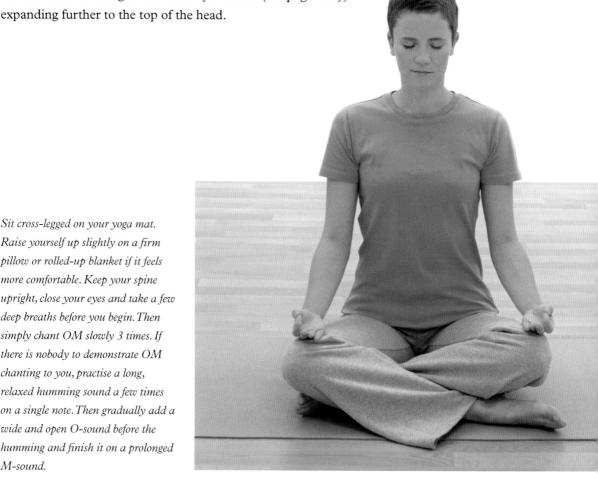

Sit cross-legged on your yoga mat. Raise yourself up slightly on a firm pillow or rolled-up blanket if it feels more comfortable. Keep your spine upright, close your eyes and take a few deep breaths before you begin. Then simply chant OM slowly 3 times. If there is nobody to demonstrate OM chanting to you, practise a long, relaxed humming sound a few times on a single note. Then gradually add a wide and open O-sound before the humming and finish it on a prolonged M-sound.

EYE EXERCISES

The involuntary muscles in our eyes are used constantly and therefore deserve specific attention and rest at times. The Eye Exercises that follow help to strengthen and improve eyesight, relax perception and therefore calm the mind.

It is best to sit cross-legged to do these exercises, with your hands loosely on your knees and your back straight so that you can breathe freely into the abdomen. There is no need to move your head, back or neck to do them, as it is all about training specific muscle groups (your eye muscles) while keeping the rest of the body motionless and relaxed. This capacity will help you to develop a relaxed awareness in all situations in life. Simply progress through all the exercises in order to give your eyes a full work-out.

During this set of exercises, it is not the focusing of the eyes that is important; it is the gentle yet firm movement of the eyes in the various directions.

Caution

Before you start this exercise, it is best to remove your glasses or hard contact lenses. You can keep soft lenses in as they will not interfere with any of the practices.

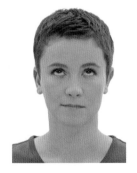
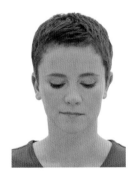

1 **Up–down** *Open your eyes wide and slowly look up and down 10 times. Then close your eyes and breathe deeply a few times. Feel your eye muscles relaxing.*

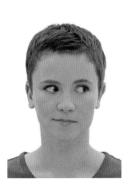
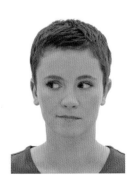

2 **Left–right** *Open your eyes again and look to the left and right 10 times. Then close your eyes, breathe deeply and relax.*

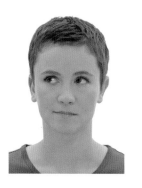

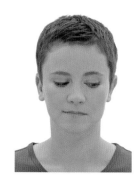

3 Diagonal *Open your eyes and look to the upper left and then lower right 10 times; close your eyes. Then look to the upper right followed by the lower left 10 times; close your eyes. Breathe deeply and relax.*

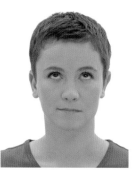

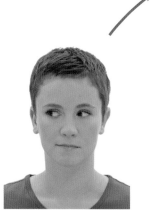

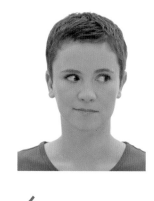

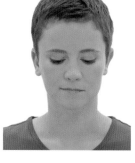

4 Circling *Open your eyes and slowly rotate them in a clockwise direction – first look up, then to the right, then down, and finally to the left. Repeat 10 times, then close your eyes and relax. Practise the same exercise counterclockwise before closing your eyes.*

5 Finishing *Rub your hands firmly together until they are warm. Then gently cup your hands over your closed eyes and let the warmth and darkness relax them.*

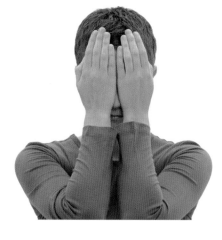

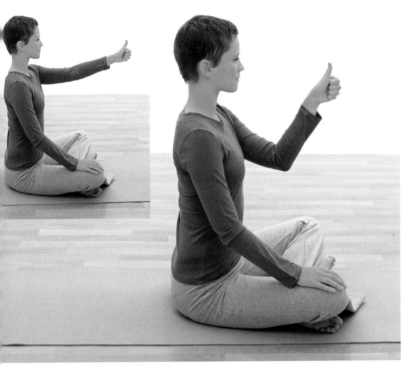

Progressive Eye-focusing

1 *Remain in a cross-legged position, with your back straight. Raise one arm in front of you, keeping your elbow straight, making a fist and raising your thumb to eye level. Focus your gaze on the tip of your thumb.*

2 *While maintaining this focus, slowly bend your arm, bringing your hand closer to your face, without losing focus. If your vision becomes blurred or your thumb appears double, this means that your hand is too close to your face. Repeat this sequence up to 5 times. Then close your eyes, breathe deeply and relax.*

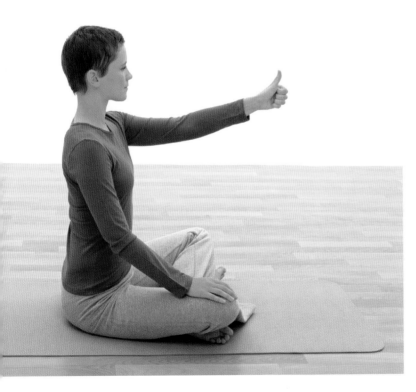

Changing Eye Focus

Remain in a cross-legged position and again extend one arm in front of you, raising your thumb to eye level. Keeping your arm fully extended, focus firstly on your thumb and then on a spot on the wall in front of you, or on the horizon. Slowly alternate this focus 10 times. Then close your eyes, breathe deeply and relax. Next, open your eyes and alternate the focus slowly between three points: the thumb, the wall or horizon and the tip of your nose. Repeat 5 times. Then close your eyes, breathe deeply and relax. Rub your hands firmly, put them over your eyes and relax.

Finish by lying down on your back in Corpse Pose to rest for 1 minute, as in Initial Relaxation (see pages 28–29).

NECK EXERCISES

The following gentle neck movements help to relieve the tension that most people hold in their neck and upper back area. It is best to sit comfortably in a cross-legged position to do the exercises – on a firm pillow or folded blanket, if desired, for comfort. Place your hands on your knees and keep your back straight to allow the breath to move freely in the abdomen. Be sure to move your head slowly throughout, keeping your eyes open.

1 *Forward–backwards* *Keeping your back straight, drop your head forward until your chin is close to your chest, letting go of its weight completely until you feel a release of tension in your neck muscles. Then move your head as far backwards as is possible, but not so much that you experience any resistance, pain or dizziness. Keep your mouth closed throughout to allow a better stretch in your throat area. Repeat this 2 times.*

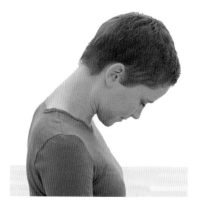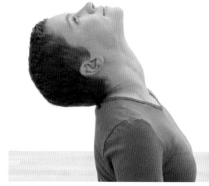

2 *Tilting right–left* *Keeping your back straight and your shoulders level, gently tilt your head to the right, bringing your ear close to your shoulder. Enjoy the stretch. Then tilt your head to the left. Repeat 2 more times on each side.*

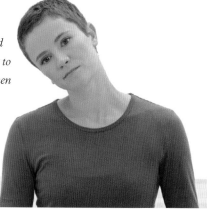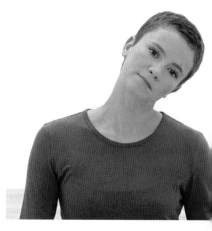

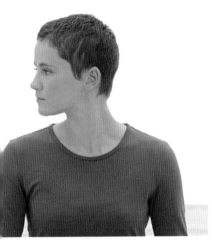

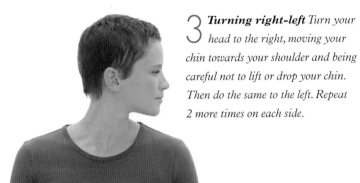

3 **Turning right-left** *Turn your head to the right, moving your chin towards your shoulder and being careful not to lift or drop your chin. Then do the same to the left. Repeat 2 more times on each side.*

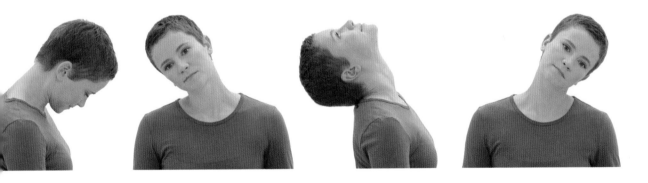

4 **Full rotation** *This is a combination of Steps 1 and 2. Keeping your back straight, drop your head forwards, then rotate it to the right, bringing your ear (not your chin) close to the shoulder, drop it back as far as you are able to without forcing it, tilt it to the left with your ear close to your shoulder and then drop it forwards again. Repeat 2 more times. Then repeat this 3 times in the opposite direction.*

Finally, lie down in Corpse Pose for 1 minute, breathing gently and practise Active Relaxation (see pages 36–37).

ACTIVE RELAXATION

It may feel as though there is no muscle effort involved in holding the body in the relaxation posture known as Corpse Pose: lying on your back as in the Initial Relaxation (see pages 28–29). Yet below our level of perception, many muscles are still slightly contracted while in the posture, which in turn maintains stress in the nervous system and depletes the body's energy levels.

Short active muscle contractions, followed by sudden and complete muscular release, will remove many of the remaining tensions, so it is a good idea to use the following active relaxation each time you enter Corpse Pose. It should only take about a minute in total.

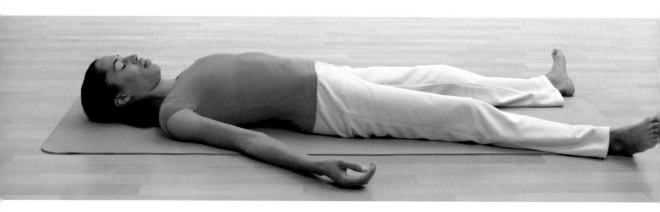

1 *Lie flat on your back, with your arms and legs slightly apart and relaxed.*

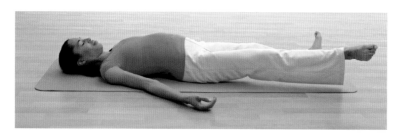

2 *Inhale deeply, lift your right leg about 5 cm (2 in) off the floor, hold your breath for a moment and focus on the muscle contraction as you resist the pull of gravity. Then exhale and drop your leg back into Corpse Pose. Take a slow breath and feel the deeper level of relaxation in your leg muscles. Inhale and repeat on the left side.*

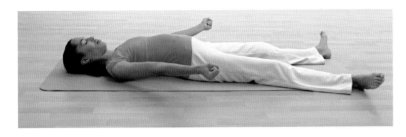

3 Inhale deeply, clench your fists and lift your arms slightly off the floor. Hold your breath, then exhale and drop your arms to the floor. Then lift your arms again, this time opening your hands and stretching your fingers wide apart. Drop your arms again and relax.

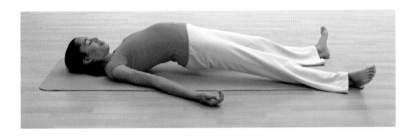

4 Inhale, contract your buttocks and lift them slightly off the floor. Hold your breath, exhale and drop your buttocks to the floor again.

5 Inhale and push your chest up, bringing your shoulder blades closer together. Hold the breath, then exhale and release your upper back to the floor.

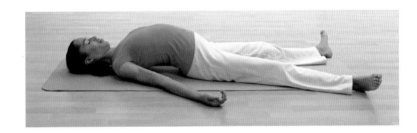

6 Inhale and pull your shoulders up and forwards, towards your ears, allowing your arms to slide along the floor. Hold your breath, tense your shoulder muscles, then exhale and release your shoulders to a relaxed position.

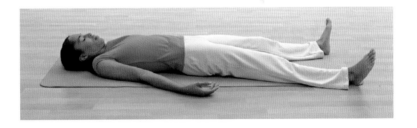

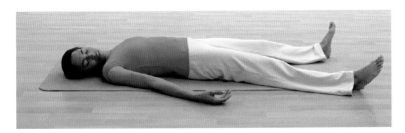

7 Inhale and gently roll your head to one side. As you exhale, turn it to the other side. Repeat several times. Your head should remain on the floor throughout the movement. Keep your chin tucked slightly towards your throat the whole time, to allow your neck to relax more.

ABDOMINAL BREATHING

Conscious control of the breath is the key to realizing all the benefits of any asana. The harmonious coordination of inhalation and exhalation creates a wave-like motion of effort and release in the nervous system, which leaves you feeling more relaxed and energetic both in body and mind after just a few minutes.

There are three main types of breathing: abdominal, chest and clavicular breathing. For now, we are concerned principally with abdominal breathing, which is essential to ventilate the major part of the lungs. On each inhalation, the diaphragm contracts and moves down against the abdominal organs, pushing the stomach out and drawing air down to the bottom of the lungs; and on each exhalation, the abdomen moves back in as the diaphragm relaxes, gently pushing against the base of the lungs and squeezing the air out.

Re-learning abdominal breathing

As abdominal breathing allows the greatest ventilation of the lungs, you might logically conclude that most people use this type of basic breathing all the time. In fact most people practise only

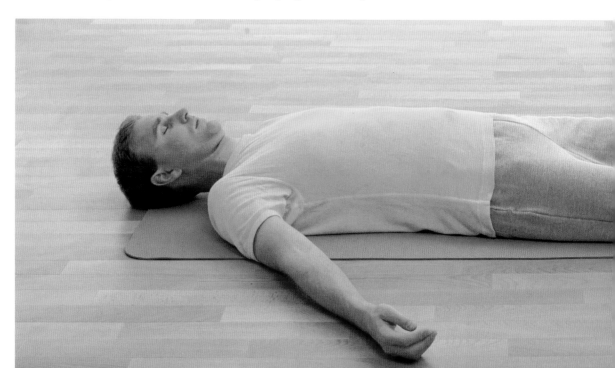

chest and clavicular breathing in daily life – even doctors and professional athletes. What is strange about this is the fact that abdominal breathing is the most natural type of breathing: children generally breathe with their abdomen, and both children and adults breathe abdominally during sleep. So what causes the body to lose this natural ability for abdominal breathing during waking adult life?

The main reason is simply stress. When you become stressed, the solar plexus (located in your abdomen), which is a major control centre for the nervous system, becomes tense, as do the abdominal muscles, which then prevents the natural movement of the diaphragm. Another reason may be fixed mental images, such as the concept of 'manhood' projecting a body position in which the chest is expanded and the abdomen tight.

Devoting a little time and attention to developing the habit of abdominal breathing will add a relaxed and dynamic quality both to your yoga practice and to your daily life. During the first few weeks of yoga practice, you may find it hard to become aware of your breathing and abdominal movement. It may therefore be helpful to practise Preparation 1 before doing the Abdominal Breathing technique itself. You may also need to do Preparation 2 occasionally before the full technique to bring your full focus to the movement of the diaphragm. However, every time you enter Corpse Pose, you should carry out abdominal breathing.

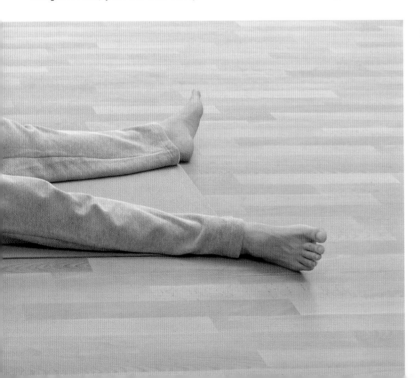

Abdominal Breathing Technique

Lie on your back in Corpse Pose, with your arms and legs apart and relaxed. Breathe in and out deeply into your abdomen for about 1 minute, being aware of your abdomen expanding as you inhale and deflating as you exhale. This may require concentration at first, but with practice it will become perfectly natural and easy.

Abdominal Breathing Preparations

The following exercises are designed to help you to
become more physically aware of your breathing
patterns, so that you can choose when you want
to breathe abdominally.

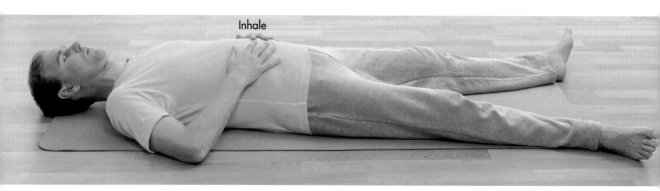

Inhale

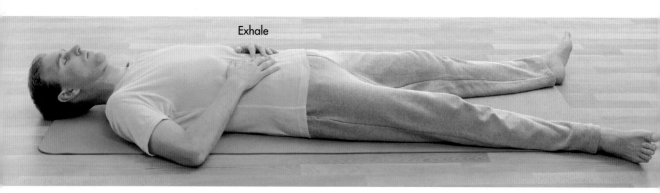

Exhale

PREPARATION 1

*Lie on your back, with your arms and
legs apart. Place your hands over your
abdomen and spread your fingers so
that you can cover the area between
your first rib and the pelvis. Breathe in
rhythmically through your nose for
2–3 seconds and out again for 2–3
seconds. Each time you inhale, feel your
abdomen rising and each time you
exhale, feel your abdomen descending.
Continue this for 1 minute.*

PREPARATION 2

1 *Place a weight (for example a book, folded towel or small cushion) on your abdomen and release your arms onto the floor in Corpse Pose. Continue breathing rhythmically and notice how your abdomen pushes the weight upwards during inhalation and relaxes downwards during exhalation. Continue this for 1 minute.*

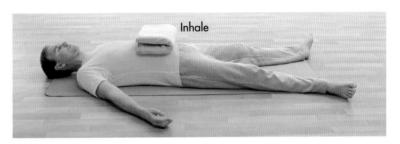

Inhale

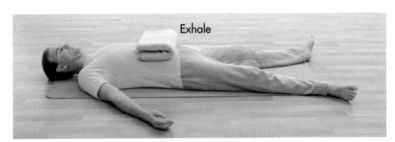

Exhale

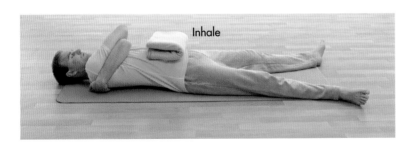

Inhale

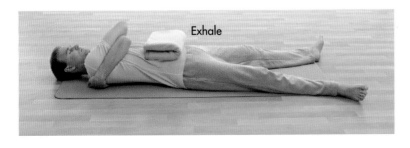

Exhale

2 *Keeping the weight on your abdomen, cross your arms tightly over your chest and try to reach your shoulder blades. This pressure on your ribcage will automatically shift your attention to abdominal breathing. Try not to let your chest move at all as you inhale, but allow your abdomen to expand more and more. Then let your abdomen come down as you exhale. Continue this for 1 minute.*

SINGLE LEG LIFTS

Regular practice of Single Leg Lifts helps to overcome muscle stiffness in the calf and hamstring muscles. These muscles often become reduced in length, causing tightness, due to lifestyle factors such as sitting on a chair all day at work. Single Leg Lifts are therefore a great way to gently stretch and warm up for a complete yoga session. If you are finding the Simple Leg Lifts too challenging at first, try the Bent-leg Adaptation. Once you become confident with this and Simple Leg Lifts, you may wish to practise the more advanced Leg-stretching Variation too.

Simple Leg Lifts

1 *Lie on your back with your legs together, arms by your sides and palms facing down.*

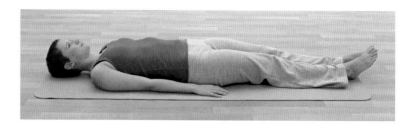

2 *Gently flex your right foot and contract the muscles around your right knee to help to keep your leg straight throughout the exercise. As you inhale for three seconds, lift your right leg to an angle of 90 degrees, then exhale and lower the leg to the same count. Avoid pressing your other leg or the palms of your hands into the floor, instead using your abdominal* *muscles to lift the leg. On your next inhalation, repeat with your left leg. Alternate sides 5 times in total. While trying to lift the leg higher each time, also focus on coordinating your breath with the movement.*

Then rest and relax in Corpse Pose for about 1 minute, as per the Relaxation Between Exercises on pages 46–47.

Bent-leg Adaptation

If you have tense back muscles or a sensitive lower back, you might find this adaptation useful to practise at first instead of the Simple Leg Lifts as it provides a more nurturing stretch.

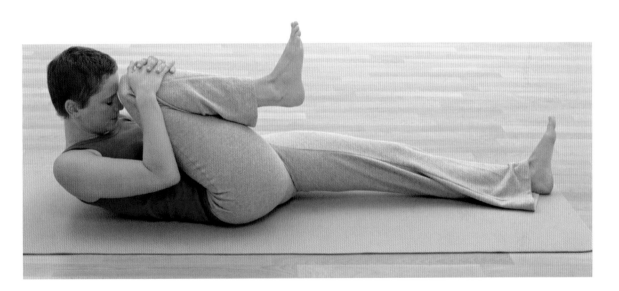

Lie comfortably on your back with your legs together and your arms at your side, palms facing down. Inhale and lift your right leg as high as is comfortable to a count of three seconds. Then exhale slowly for three, bend your right leg towards your chest, wrap your arms around your

bent knee and firmly pull it into your abdomen. Maintaining this pressure, take a deep abdominal inhalation, and lift your head, bringing your forehead as close to your knee as possible. Then exhale and release your head, leg and arms to the floor. Repeat with your left leg. Alternate sides 5 times in total.

Then finish with Relaxation Between Exercises in Corpse Pose (see pages 46–47).

Leg-stretching Variation

This is a more challenging stretching exercise and should
only be attempted once you are completely comfortable
with the Simple Leg Lifts. If you do it slowly, regularly
and with deep abdominal breathing, the stretching gradually
becomes easier and your leg muscles will start to lengthen.

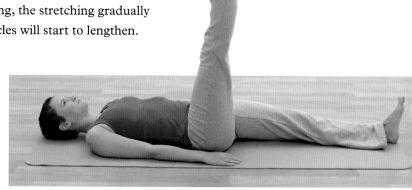

1 *Lie on your back with your legs
together and arms at your side,
palms facing down. Inhale for a count
of three and lift your right leg as high
as you can, with your foot flexed and
your leg completely straight.*

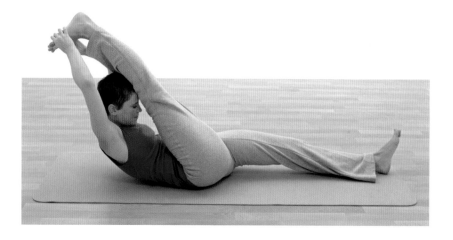

2 *As you exhale for three,
take hold of your leg as
high as you can with both
hands, without allowing it to
bend. Still on this exhalation,
lift your back and try to
bring your forehead as close
as possible to your knee.*

3 *As you inhale, lower your back
and head to the floor, keeping a
firm grip on your leg and creating a
strong stretch along the full length of
your leg. Exhale and slowly lower your
leg and arms to the floor. Then repeat
this sequence on the left leg. Alternate
between legs 5 times in total.*

*Finish with Relaxation Between
Exercises in Corpse Pose for about
1 minute (see pages 46–47).*

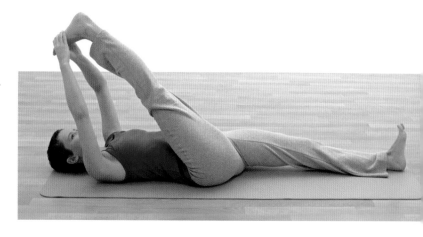

Muscle stretching

The general rule for any yoga exercise is that if you experience a painful reaction anywhere in the body, you should immediately reduce or stop the exercise and relax on your back. When it comes to muscle stretching, however, the body's natural reaction is a certain amount of muscle discomfort at first – especially if you are not used to exercising in this way. It may require some practice to distinguish between this 'stretch discomfort' from the discomfort or pain caused by other, negative factors, such as a compressed nerve. The best way to observe the difference is to see how the pain reacts to rest and deep and rhythmical abdominal breathing: stretch pain will subside quickly, whereas another type of pain may not.

If you find a certain muscle stretch uncomfortable, it is advisable to hold it only for a few breaths and then return to Corpse Pose (see pages 28–29). The pain should dissolve after resting with a few deep abdominal breaths and you will feel pleasantly warm and relaxed. Once you are more experienced, you will learn how to breathe the discomfort away while continuing to stretch the muscle. It requires a lot of patience and discrimination to deal with your body's reactions.

THE BENEFITS OF STRETCHING

Typical starting scenario	Improvement through yoga
General fatigue: the exercise seems demanding and tiring	Deep abdominal breathing increases vitality and removes fatigue
Body and mind are under stress; muscle stretch is painful and stressful	Repeated muscle stretching and relaxation activates the rest and repair process in the nervous system; resistance to stress increases
Muscles are stiff; stretching is difficult; muscles shorten and stiffen further the next day	Less resistance in the muscles during stretching; quick release of stretch discomfort with rhythmical abdominal breathing; regaining natural flexibility on a permanent basis

RELAXATION BETWEEN EXERCISES

It is important to rest in Corpse Pose after every exercise for a number of reasons. First and foremost, it allows you to recuperate from the effort of the previous exercise and helps to avoid any build-up of lactic acid, which may lead to muscle fatigue. However, it also gives you an opportunity to observe how the benefits of each exercise are being absorbed by the body, as well as providing a well-balanced rhythm of exercise and relaxation. It is best to allow between 30 seconds and 2 minutes for this relaxation process.

1 *Lie on your back in Corpse Pose, with your arms and legs slightly apart. Apply all or any of the active relaxation movements in Steps 2–7, depending on which parts of the body were involved in the most recent exercise (see also pages 36–37).*

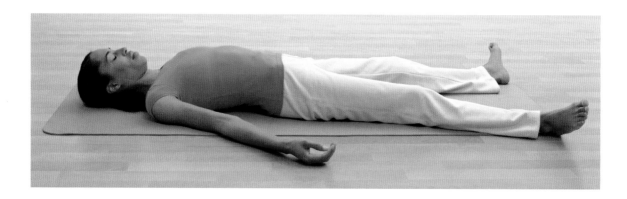

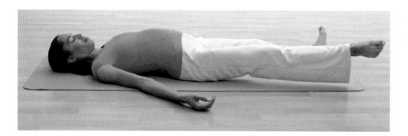

2 *Raise one leg at a time and drop it.*

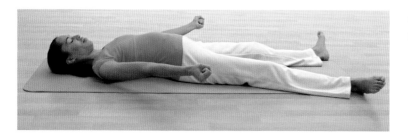

3 *Clench your fists, raise both arms and drop them.*

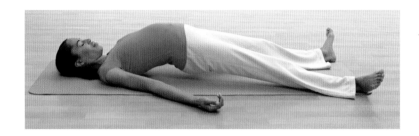

4 *Lift your hips and release them.*

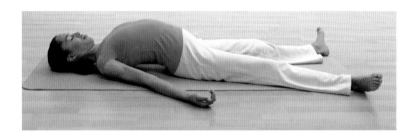

5 *Lift your chest and release it.*

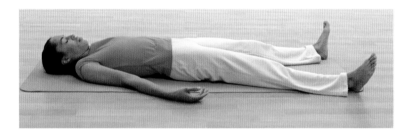

6 *Pull your shoulders up to your ears and release them.*

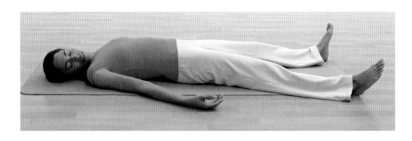

7 *Slowly roll your head from side to side.*

Remaining in Corpse Pose, take three deep breaths. Then continue with slow, rhythmical abdominal breathing for about 1 minute (see pages 38–41) and try to relax your body from your feet up to your head, focusing on the parts where most of the muscle stretch or contraction has just occurred.

DOUBLE LEG LIFTS

These leg-lifting exercises really strengthen the abdominal muscles. They are therefore excellent for developing good postural alignment and for correcting postural problems, such as hyperlordosis (exaggerated lumbar curvature). Abdominal strength is also important for the practice of certain asanas, such as Half Headstand (see pages 120–123) and Headstand (see pages 126–127). Feel free to do whichever adaptation suits you best until you feel confident and comfortable enough to do Full Double Leg Lifts.

Caution

If you suffer from sciatic pain, you should not attempt any Double Leg Lifts. Instead, do the Bent-leg Adaptation of Single Leg Lifts (see page 43). Then, once the sciatica improves, you might wish to try the Bent-leg Adaptation of Double Leg Lifts.

Full Double Leg Lifts

1 *Lie on your back with your legs together and your arms at your sides, palms facing down. Tuck your chin slightly towards your throat so that the back of your neck is extended.*

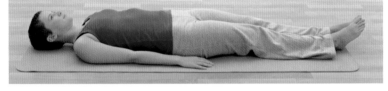

2 *As you inhale, start contracting your abdominal muscles while your legs remain on the floor. Continue the inhalation for 3 seconds, as you flex your feet and lift your legs, parallel to one another, as far towards a 90-degree angle with the floor as you can manage. Then exhale to a count of three, slowly lowering your legs back to the floor. Repeat up to 9 more times, slowly.*

Relax in Corpse Pose for about 1 minute before the next posture (see pages 46–47).

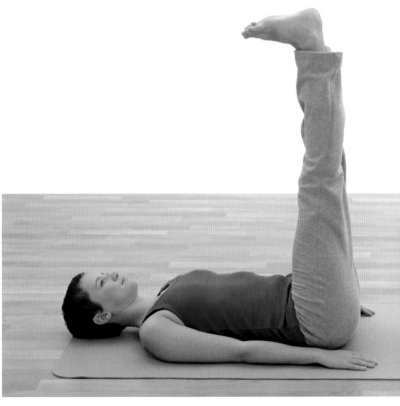

Double Leg Lift Adaptations

In the beginning you may experience a few difficulties with the full exercise if your abdominal muscles are a little weak. For example, while lifting your legs, your lower back might move away from the floor, you might feel pressure or discomfort in your lower back or your shoulders may become tense. If you have any of these difficulties, experiment to discover which of the following adaptations suits you best.

STABILITY ADAPTATION

If your lower back hurts when lifting your legs, place your arms under your body for stability, with your hands under your buttocks and your palms facing down. Then do Steps 1 and 2 as in the main exercise.

BENT-LEG ADAPTATION

Do Steps 1 and 2 as in the main exercise, but allow your legs to bend when lifting and lowering them, removing the pressure on your lower back. Unfortunately, however, this greatly reduces the work-out for the abdominal muscles.*

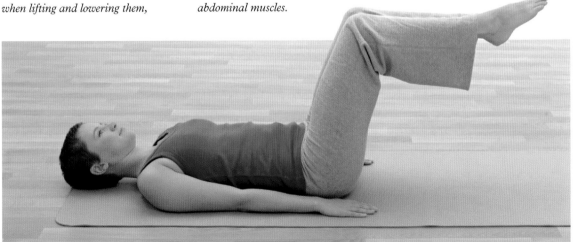

SHOULDERSTAND

Sarvangasana

The Sanskrit name of this inverted pose, *Sarvangasana*, means 'posture for all parts of the body'. The change in circulation that it causes (increased blood supply to the brain), as well as the balancing effect it has on the thyroid gland (which helps to govern metabolism), means that this asana can restore vitality to the mind and body in just a matter of minutes. It also mobilizes the upper spine and shoulder joints, strengthens the lower back and arms, and releases stress and tension via the thorough stretch it gives the spine.

Basic Shoulderstand

1 *Lie on your back with your legs together and your arms on the floor, close to the body, palms facing down.*

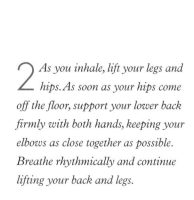

2 *As you inhale, lift your legs and hips. As soon as your hips come off the floor, support your lower back firmly with both hands, keeping your elbows as close together as possible. Breathe rhythmically and continue lifting your back and legs.*

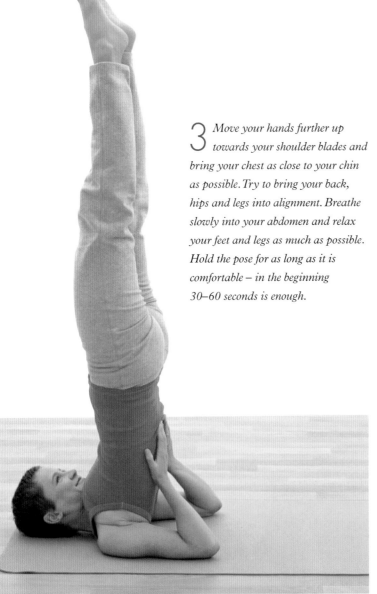

3 *Move your hands further up towards your shoulder blades and bring your chest as close to your chin as possible. Try to bring your back, hips and legs into alignment. Breathe slowly into your abdomen and relax your feet and legs as much as possible. Hold the pose for as long as it is comfortable – in the beginning 30–60 seconds is enough.*

4 *To release the pose, lower both arms to the floor, pressing them firmly into the ground for balance. Slightly bend at the waist and then roll down vertebra by vertebra, using your arms as a brake. Once your pelvis is touching the floor use your abdominal muscles to lower your legs slowly to the floor.*

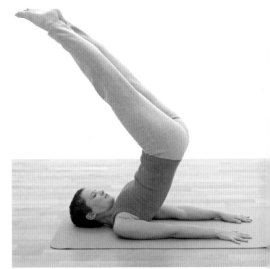

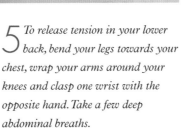

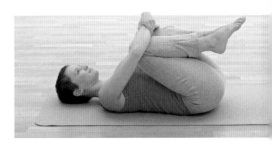

5 *To release tension in your lower back, bend your legs towards your chest, wrap your arms around your knees and clasp one wrist with the opposite hand. Take a few deep abdominal breaths.*

Then release your arms and legs to rest and relax in Final Relaxation (see pages 54–57).

FINAL RELAXATION

This relaxation is the most rewarding moment of the session. It increases the benefits of each asana and brings your body and mind into a state of perfect balance via relaxation on three levels: physical, mental and spiritual. Allow 10–15 minutes for the sequence. Just as the movement or contraction of a muscle requires a thought process to make it happen, so does the relaxation of a muscle. The Relaxation Pose, or Corpse Pose, does not require any actual physical effort, which means you can pay full attention to simply relaxing all the muscles and organs for a change.

Physical relaxation

In order to relax all the muscles in your body, focus one last time on a very active contraction of the muscles. This is similar to the Active Relaxation movements that you have been practising between exercises, but there are also a few new facial movements and you should hold each muscle contraction for a little longer. It is advised to contract your muscles as you inhale hold it for 2–3 seconds and then relax completely as you exhale.

1 *Lie flat on your back in Corpse Pose, with your arms and legs slightly apart.*

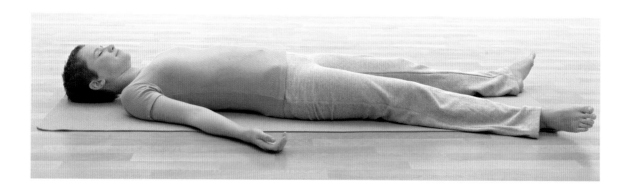

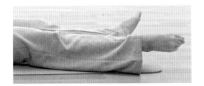

2 *Lift your right leg about 5 cm (2 in) off the floor and drop it back down. Then repeat on the left leg.*

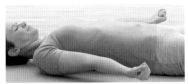

3 *Lift both your arms, clench your fists, then drop your arms and release the fingers.*

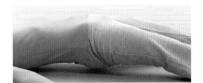

4 *Contract your buttocks to lift your hips off the floor, then release them.*

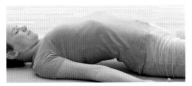

5 *Lift your chest off the floor, pushing it high, then release it.*

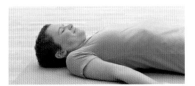

6 *Pull your shoulders tightly up to your ears, then release them.*

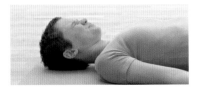

7 *Contract all your facial muscles towards your nose, then release them.*

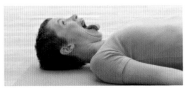

8 *Open your mouth, stick out your tongue, open your eyes wide and look upwards to give your facial muscles a full stretch. Then release.*

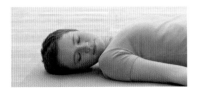

9 *Slowly roll your head from side to side, making sure that your arms and legs are still slightly apart and away from your body.*

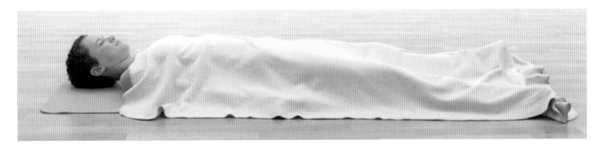

10 *Cover yourself with a light blanket to keep warm. This is especially important for people who have low blood pressure as they may feel slightly cold as the relaxation progresses. Watch your abdomen rising with each inhalation and lowering with each exhalation, and observe the gentle air flow in the nostrils. Now start sending a clear message to your feet: 'I am relaxing my feet, I am relaxing my feet, my feet are relaxed.' Continue sending similar 'autosuggestion' messages to your various body parts until you reach your head. Once you have relaxed all the muscles, send positive messages to your internal organs: 'I am relaxing my kidneys, I am relaxing my kidneys, my kidneys are relaxed.' Continue with all other organs, including the brain at the end. With practice, you will actually feel your internal organs relaxing and recharging as you do this.*

Class 2

Class 2 builds on what you have already learned in Class 1, introducing deep yogic breathing and Sun Salutation, which stretches all the major muscles of the body. You may notice that after this dynamic warm-up sequence, your body adjusts quite easily to the new asanas that follow: the Plough, the Fish, Forward Bend, Inclined Plane, the Cobra and Child's Pose. This is because your body naturally enters a deeper level of relaxation once you have practised a sequence of forward bends and backbends, or poses and counter-poses.

How are you doing with the regularity of your practice? It is important to remember that doing a little regularly is best. Try to practise at least every other day, if possible. To help you to integrate the practice into your daily schedule, Classes 2–8 offer the possibility of doing a shortened practice when you do not have time to complete the whole class. This is how it works: the exercises of one session are identified by a circle symbol ● and those of the other session are identified by a triangle symbol ▲. Both sessions are complete yoga work-outs in their own right. Exercises that need to be done in all sessions are identified with both symbols ● ▲.

How long does the class take?

15 minutes to read through the class
50–60 minutes to practise it for the first time
40–50 minutes when repeating the practice

Practice for busy people in 2 separate sessions (30–40 minutes):
Session A ●
Session B ▲

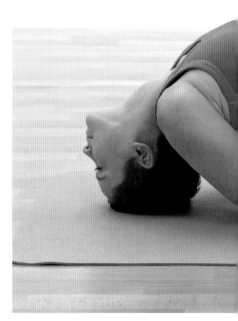

EXERCISE PLAN

❋ Indicates a new exercise

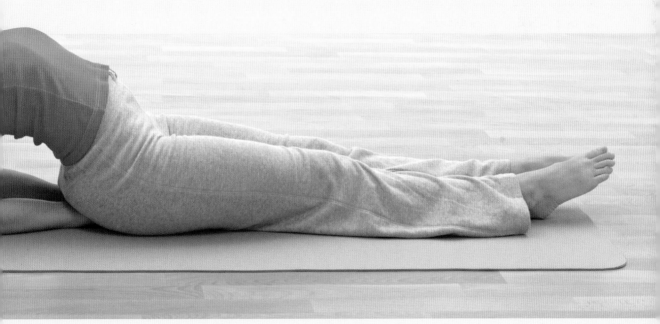

COMPLETE YOGIC BREATH

In most cases, deep breathing happens only during strenuous, physical activity, such as while doing an aerobic sport or climbing steep stairs. At that time, the increased muscular effort requires greater amounts of oxygen and the autonomic (involuntary) nervous system therefore activates a deeper and faster breath. Yet it is not the skeletal muscles that require the greatest amount of oxygen; it is, in fact, the brain. If the brain does not receive enough oxygen, its mental efficiency reduces drastically.

In today's society, most people have mind-based occupations (rather than physical ones), yet the typical work routine consists of sitting at a desk, where the flow of fresh air is minimal and optimal breathing is difficult. Besides taking regular breaks and trying to simply breathe deeply, Complete Yogic Breath is an excellent way of increasing your mental efficiency at work. Whenever you feel mentally tired at work, practise each of the following exercises for a minute or two and you will soon feel revitalized.

Complete Yogic Breath entails using all three sets of respiratory muscles – those in the abdomen, chest and clavicle (collarbone). This allows you to use your lungs to their full capacity and increase the oxygen intake to all your body's cells. Although chest breathing allows a considerable increase of vital capacity, it is actually the abdominal breath that fills the greatest part of the lungs. Clavicular breathing is the final part of Complete Yogic Breath. On its own, it is not very meaningful as it fills only a very small part of the top of the lungs, but as part of the whole sequence it completes the full expansion of the chest and is an excellent means of overcoming rounded shoulders. Notice how the extra oxygen you gain from Complete Yogic Breath refreshes your mind and improves your sensory perception.

Deepening the abdominal breath

1 *Lie down in Corpse Pose (see page 28) and place both hands on your abdomen, with your fingers wide apart. Your thumbs should touch your first ribs and your little fingers should touch your hip bones. While inhaling and exhaling to a count of three seconds each, notice how your whole abdomen expands and contracts rhythmically. Continue this for 1 minute. Then lower your arms back to the floor in Relaxation Pose.*

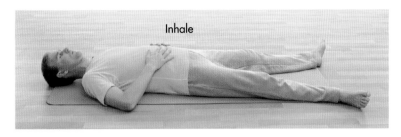

Inhale

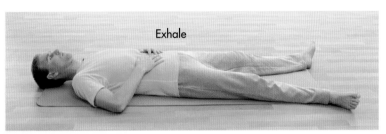

Exhale

2 *Now sit cross-legged and practise the same abdominal breathing exercise for 1 minute. You may need to sit on a small cushion to keep your spine in an upright position without too much effort.*

3 *Next, practise it in a standing position, with your legs slightly apart, for 1 minute.*

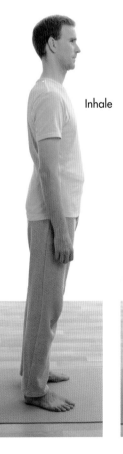

Inhale

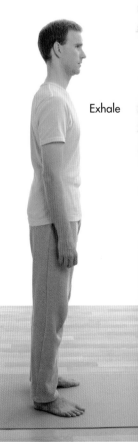

Exhale

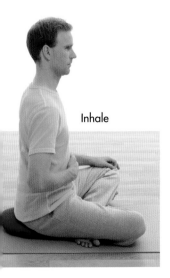

Inhale

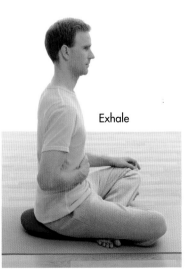

Exhale

Adding chest breathing

1 *Lie down in Corpse Pose, place one hand on your abdomen and the other on your chest. After a complete abdominal inhalation (allowing your abdomen to expand), continue inhaling by lifting and expanding your ribcage.*

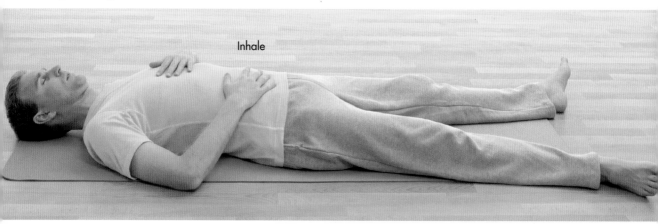

Inhale

2 *Then begin exhaling from your abdomen, followed immediately by the release of the intercostal muscles between the ribs, bringing your chest back to its resting position. As you increase the length and depth of the*

breath, make sure that your abdomen remains expanded when you add the chest breathing, and that the exhalation always starts from your abdomen, before your chest. Continue this for about 1 minute.

Then practise the same type of breathing sitting cross-legged for 1 minute and, next, in a standing position for 1 minute.

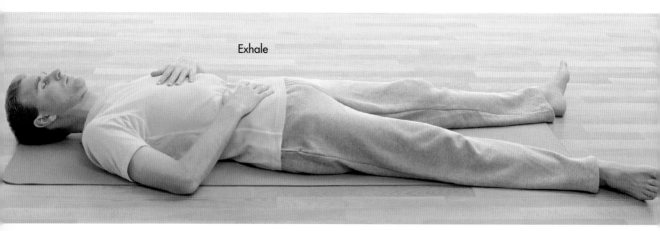

Exhale

Adding clavicular breathing

1 *Again, lie down in Corpse Pose and place one hand on your abdomen and the other on your chest. After a complete inhalation into your abdomen and chest, try to fill the very top of your lungs by lifting your collarbone (clavicle). Make sure that your abdomen remains expanded and that you are not pulling your shoulders up to your ears, as this would have no effect on your lung capacity.*

2 *Then begin the exhalation from your abdomen, immediately followed by releasing the air from your chest and clavicle area. Continue this for about 1 minute.*

3 *Next, try to practise this sitting in front of a mirror, so that you can actually see the contraction of the muscles on each side of your throat (called sternocleidomastoid muscles).*

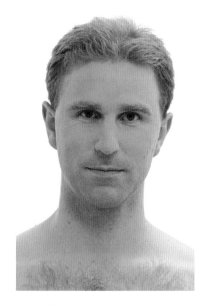

Normal breathing

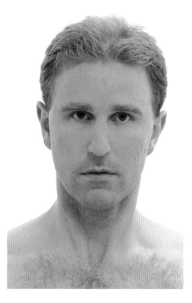

Clavicular breathing

Applying Complete Yogic Breath

Every time you relax between exercises, start with 3–5 Complete Yogic Breaths. The extra oxygen will allow the muscles to relax faster. As the complete respiratory movement begins from below the waist and reaches up to the neck area, it will also help to balance your spinal position. After 3–5 Complete Yogic Breaths, continue the usual abdominal breathing, inhaling to a count of three seconds and exhaling to a count of three seconds.

5 *Holding your breath, bring your left leg back into push-up-position and look straight ahead. This does not necessarily mean that you have to look to the front; it simply means that you should follow your* *natural line of vision when your neck is in line with your spine, so check that your body and neck are in a straight line. You may want to lower and lift your hips a few times until you find the correct alignment.*

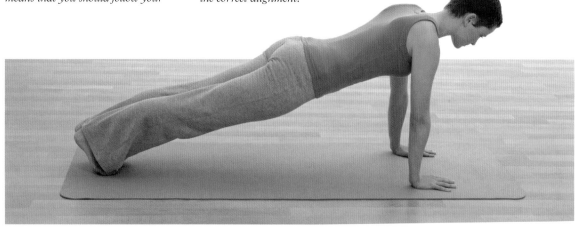

6 *As you exhale, gradually bend your knees and lower your chest and forehead to the floor, but keep your hips off the floor.*

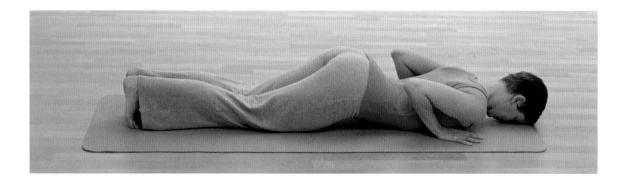

7 *As you inhale, lie flat on the floor, stretch your toes (so that the tops of your feet are on the floor), slowly lift your head and chest, and look up. Besides pushing with your arms, use the muscles of your neck and upper back to lift you. This will help you to avoid putting too much pressure on your lower back. Your arms should remain bent.*

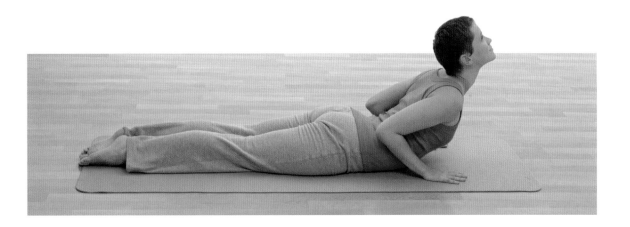

8 *As you exhale, lift your hips up and push your heels as far as possible into the floor. Do not worry if you cannot put your heels flat on the floor: this is simply due to tight hamstrings and is quite common. Do not, however, try to compensate by walking forward as this will disturb the symmetrical alignment of the next movement. Look to your feet.*

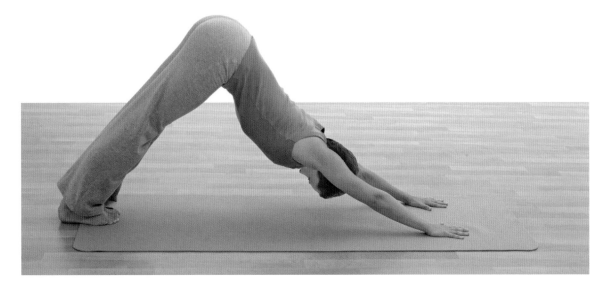

9 *As you inhale, take a large step (or lunge) forward to bring your right foot between your hands, and lower your back knee to the floor, so that the top of your back foot is on the mat. Look up.*

10 *As you exhale, bring your left leg forward, straighten both legs as much as possible and bend down until your head touches your knees. Bend your knees a little if necessary to reach this position, keeping your hands on the floor next to your feet.*

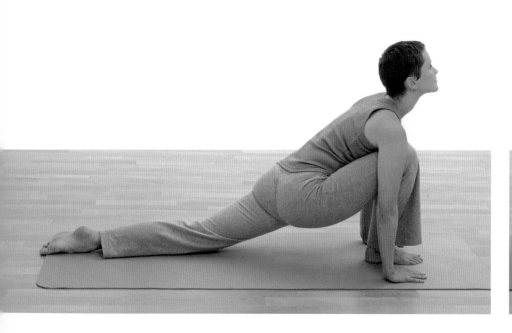

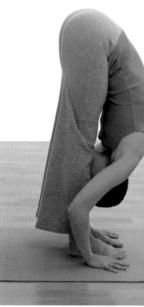

11 *As you inhale, stretch your arms forward and up, keeping your arms next to your ears. Arch back from your chest and stretch your arms and fingers.*

12 *As you exhale, return to a standing position, releasing your arms to hang by your sides. Now take a deep inhalation in this position.*

13 *Put your hands back in Prayer Position as you exhale, and start again with Step 1. This time do movements 4 and 9 with your left leg first. Repeat the whole sequence 3–5 times in total.*

Then relax in Corpse Pose, starting with a Complete Yogic Breath, until the heartbeat has returned to normal (see pages 46–47).

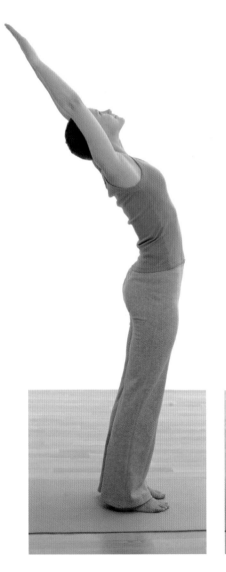

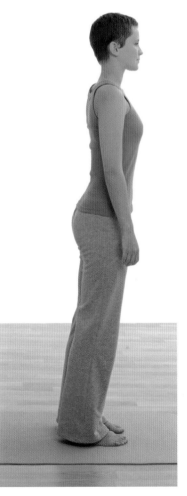

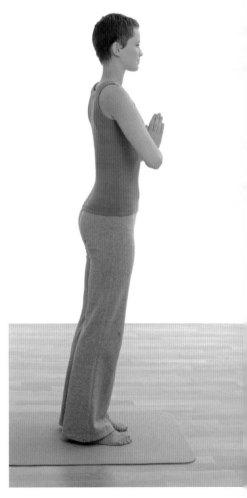

Help with Step 6

If you find Step 6 of Sun Salutation difficult, as many people do at first because it feels slightly unusual, try going into the pose from the lying position.

Lie flat on your abdomen, with your forehead and chest in a relaxed position on the floor and your toes tucked under. Now slowly walk your knees slightly closer to your chest, making sure your forehead and chest remain on the floor, allowing your hips to rise and keeping your toes tucked under. If you walk too far forward,

your hips will be too high, the pressure on your nose will become painful and your chest may lift off the floor. Once you have found a balanced position, try to reach it from push-up position: carefully lower both knees, releasing much of your body weight, and then position your chest between your hands and forehead on the floor.

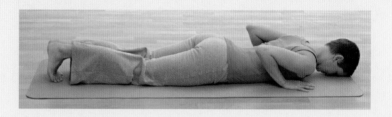

Help with Step 9

If you find it too difficult to step or lunge your foot all the way forward between your hands, then you can take the following measures.

First, lower the opposite knee slowly to the floor (see top right). Then catch the ankle of the leg you want to bring forward with one hand and gently ease the foot into position (see bottom right).

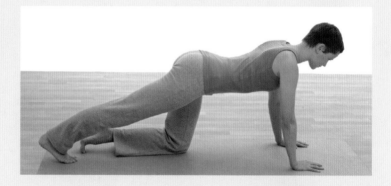

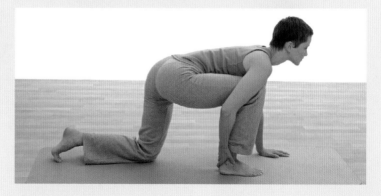

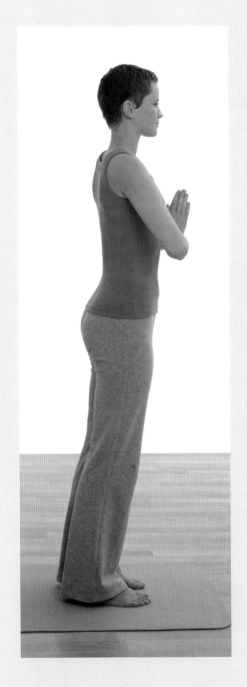

Benefits of Sun Salutation

The Sun Salutation sequence is a complete aerobic exercise in itself, largely because of the two expansive movements – from standing upright with lifted arms down to the standing forward bend and back up again. A few rounds of Sun Salutation followed by a few minutes of deep relaxation would take only ten minutes of your day and would have an invigorating yet relaxing effect on your whole being. So why not start integrating it into your daily routine in order to reap some of the many benefits that the 12 simple, flowing movements have to offer:

• The wide range of movement mobilizes the whole spine and stretches and strengthens hundreds of muscles.

• The smooth alternation between forward-bending and back-bending massages the solar plexus, which, in turn, promotes deep, abdominal breathing.

• The systematic breathing (inhaling on each backbend and exhaling on each forward bend) increases the respiratory capacity of the lungs.

• The synchronized flow of muscle contraction and release rhythmically stimulates and relaxes the nervous system, eliminating a lot of stress. The Sun Salutation sequence is therefore a good nerve tonic.

• The flowing nature of the movements in harmony with the breath promotes a state of relaxed attention.

• The sequence of movements provides a full anterior (front) and posterior (back) stretch of the body – stretching everything from your hands, arms, armpits, chest, abdomen and throat to your thigh muscles, hamstrings and back muscles.

• The varied range of movement involved in the sequence considerably enhances flexibility of the hips, pelvis, upper back, neck and shoulders.

• As well as making you feel generally more vibrant and healthy, daily Sun Salutation practice will greatly enhance your yoga practice as it warms up the entire body, improving the efficiency of your muscles throughout the asanas.

THE PLOUGH ●

Halasana

The body looks somewhat like a plough, or *hala* in Sanskrit, when in this posture. The Plough stretches the whole back of your body, mobilizing your entire spine and increasing blood supply to the spinal nerves, and the hyperextension of the arms also improves shoulder flexibility. Deep, abdominal breathing in this posture also gives a gentle massage to the abdominal organs.

1 *Lie on your back, with your legs together and your arms by your sides.*

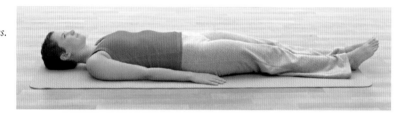

2 *As you inhale, lift your legs, pelvis and lower back, firmly supporting the back with both hands.*

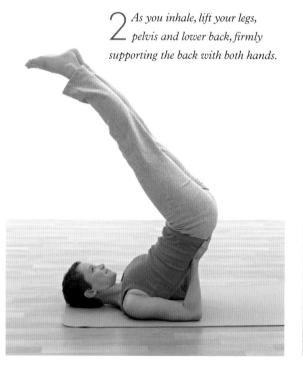

3 *Continue the movement with steady breathing, bringing your legs over your head and progressively bringing the spine to a vertical position.*

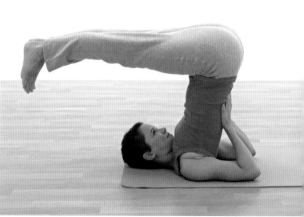

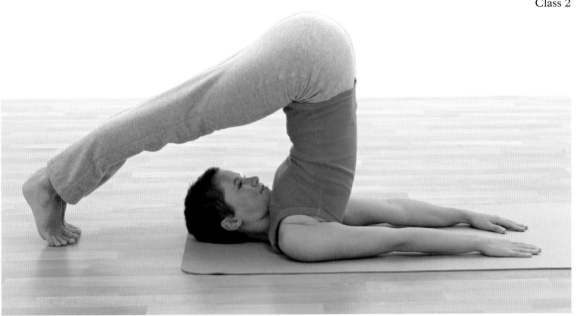

4 *Keeping your legs straight and toes flexed, stretch your feet down towards the floor behind you. If your feet touch the ground, lower* your arms to the floor behind your back. If your feet can't yet reach the floor, simply hold them in the furthest position they will go and continue to *support your back with both hands for stability. Hold the pose for up to 1 minute, with slow rhythmical breathing.*

5 *Then release the pose by rolling down vertebra by vertebra, with your arms pushing against the floor for balance.*

Relax in Corpse Pose for 1 minute (see pages 46–47) before moving into the next posture.

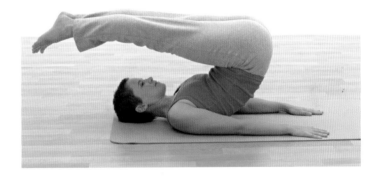

Plough adaptation

If, due to muscles tightness, your feet do not reach the floor, try opening your legs wide and bringing your arms over your head until your hands are close to your feet. Your feet may reach the floor quite easily now, in which case you should try to catch hold of your ankles or toes.

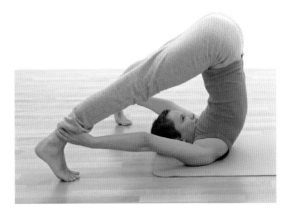

THE FISH

Matsyasana

The Fish acts as a gentle counter-pose to the Shoulderstand sequence, of which the Plough is part. After practising the Fish, you will experience a renewed sense of balance throughout your spine, encouraging deep relaxation throughout the body. The posture increases the vital capacity of the lungs, reduces bronchial congestion, brings flexibility to the upper spine, and revitalizes the thyroid gland, which governs metabolism.

The neck position

Even if you found the backwards movement of the neck difficult or painful during the Neck Exercises (see pages 34–35), you may find the same movement quite easy in the Fish posture. This is because the neck movement here is simply a natural continuation of the backwards curve of the spine.

1 *Lie down on your back, place both arms under your body, with your hands as far as possible under your thighs (palms down) and your elbows as far as possible under your back. This position pulls your shoulders further back, increasing the potential for chest curve in the movement to come.*

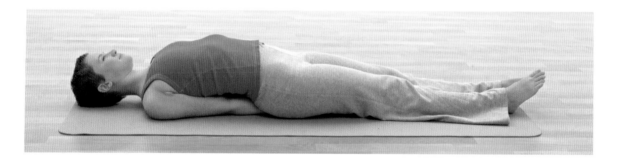

2 *As you inhale, lift your chest as high possible, bending your arms, arching your back and carefully bending your neck backwards.*

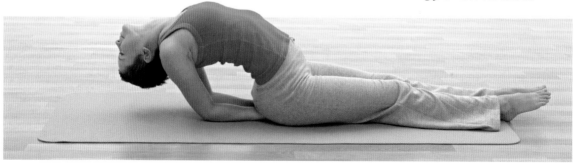

3 *Then, maintaining the arched back, slowly lower your body until the top of your head gently touches the floor. Keep most of your weight firmly on your elbows, avoiding* pressure in the neck area. For stability, hold your feet together, yet at the same time allow your legs to relax. Hold the pose for half the time spent in Shoulderstand, which in this class would mean about 30–60 seconds. Keep your mouth closed throughout to increase the stretch in your throat and chest, and practise Complete Yogic Breath (see pages 60–63).

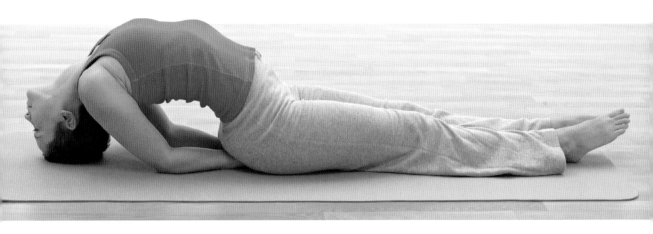

4 *To release the asana, push firmly on your elbows, lift your head slightly and lower your back to the floor.*

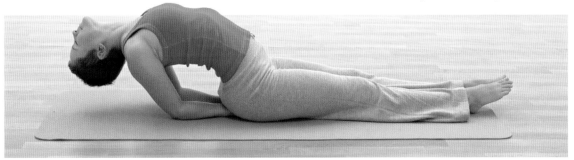

5 *As a gentle counter-stretch, place both your hands behind your head, support your head on both sides with your bent arms and lift your head up to your chest as you inhale. As you exhale, slowly lower your head to the floor.*

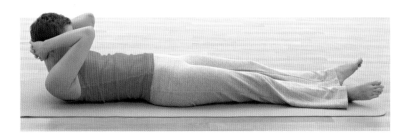

Relax in Corpse Pose for 1 minute (see pages 46–47) before moving into the next posture.

FORWARD BEND ▲

Paschimottasana

Forward Bend is a boon for many of the typical postural problems related to modern life, whereby a lot of the body's major muscles have become shortened due to stress, lack of exercise and bad postural habits, such as spending so much time sitting on chairs. By restoring flexibility to all the posterior (back) muscles of the body, Forward Bend prevents and alleviates many types of muscular tension in the back and helps to correct an exaggerated lower back curve. It also lengthens the lower back muscles and hamstrings (the muscles on the back of your upper legs), improves postural alignment and reduces nervous tension in the body.

The efficiency of the Forward Bend stretch depends mostly on keeping your legs straight and on the proper position of all ten toes, which must be pulled towards you (flexed) before lowering the body into the pose.

Smooth transition

It is important that your yoga practice flows together as smoothly as possible, so be careful how you make the transition from lying down after the Fish posture (see pages 74–75) to sitting in this posture. There are three different options you can use, depending upon how strong and flexible you are.

For strong and flexible people: Extend your arms above your head, inhale and sit up, using your abdominal muscles.

For people of medium strength and flexibility: Place your hands on your thighs, inhale and sit up.

For people with little strength and/or a sensitive lower back: Bend one leg, hold the knee with interlocked fingers, inhale and sit up by pushing the knee forward.

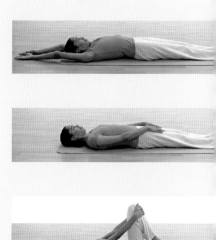

1 *Sit on your mat with both legs stretched in front of you, flex your feet, inhale and stretch both arms straight up in the air.*

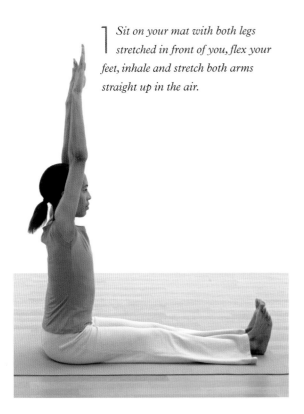

2 *Exhale and start to bend forward from the lower back, extending from the hips.*

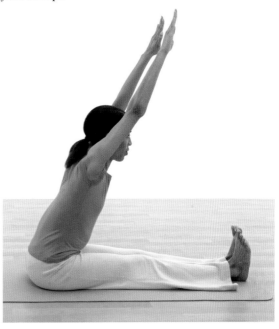

3 *Bend forward until your hands reach either your calves, ankles or feet, and reach your head and spine fowards as much as possible. Allow your elbows to hang loose to release tension in your neck and shoulders;* aim to keep your upper back, neck and head all in one line; and breathe slowly and deeply. If your hands reach your feet without compromising your straight legs, wrap your index finger around your big toe, with the thumb on top (see inset picture). This is the classical yogic foot-hold. Stay bent over here for about 1 minute before lifting the arms again and then relaxing them on an inhalation.

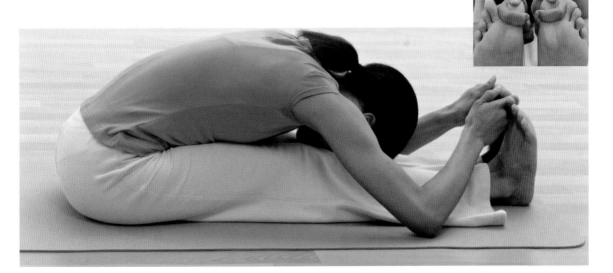

Increased-stretch Variation

Stretching the muscles near the coccyx and sacrum releases
a lot of tension and unblocks the energies in the lower spine.
However, this stretch is rarely reached in full Forward Bend
due to stiffness in the leg muscles. You may therefore like to
try the following variation.

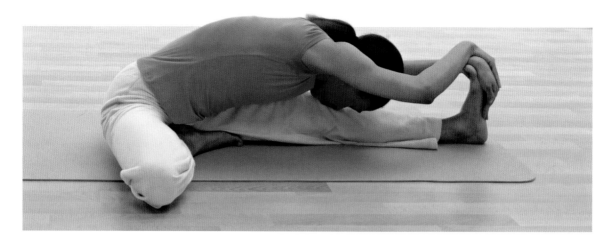

*Place your left foot against the inside
of your right thigh (as close to the
groin as possible), with your left knee
bent out to the side. Inhale, lift your
arms up and, keeping your right foot
flexed, bend over the right leg, catching
hold of either the foot, ankle or calf.
Then repeat with the opposite leg.*

Overcoming mental resistance

Even normal sitting or standing
requires contraction of the back
muscles. Therefore letting go of all
muscular contraction in the back and
allowing a full stretch of the posterior
side of the body during Forward
Bend is unusual.

You need to both physically
and mentally be able to 'let go'
of all resistance, accepting temporary
loss of control, as well as accepting
any stretch discomfort initially
created by the pose. Use rhythmical
abdominal breathing to help you
with this.

INCLINED PLANE ▲

Both length and strength are needed in the muscles for optimal mobility in all joints. After stretching the back muscles in Forward Bend, you are now going to contract the same muscles (and thus strengthen them) in Inclined Plane. An important counter-pose to Forward Bend, this posture improves your sense of balance, as well as strengthening the lower back, leg and arm muscles.

Foot cramps

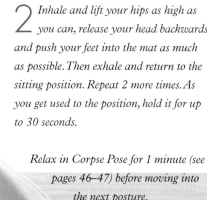

In the initial stages of your asana practice, you may occasionally experience foot cramps, especially in Inclined Plane. If a cramp occurs, sit up, breathe deeply and gently massage and move the foot around until it subsides.

1 *Sit with your legs straight out in front of you and place your hands firmly behind you on the mat, fingers pointing away from your body.*

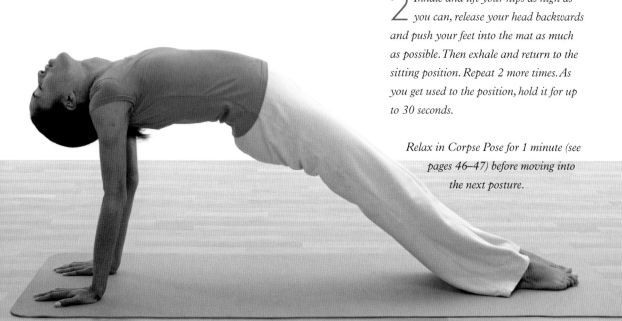

2 *Inhale and lift your hips as high as you can, release your head backwards and push your feet into the mat as much as possible. Then exhale and return to the sitting position. Repeat 2 more times. As you get used to the position, hold it for up to 30 seconds.*

Relax in Corpse Pose for 1 minute (see pages 46–47) before moving into the next posture.

THE COBRA .

Bhujangasana

Like all backbends, the Cobra greatly improves the strength and flexibility of the whole back, as well as toning the abdominal organs and muscles. The fact that you begin this one lying on your stomach allows you to increase the spinal curve very gradually, according to the strength of your back muscles. It is best to do the Half Cobra first to warm you up and then move on to the Full Basic Cobra. If you are finding these uncomfortable, try the adaptation on page 82 to start with. Whenever there is sensitivity or pain anywhere in the spine, reduce the effort and allow the spine to bend less, remaining in a comfortable zone of back extension.

Half Cobra

1 *Lie on your front, rest your forehead on the mat and place your hands next to your chest, aligning the fingertips with your shoulders.*

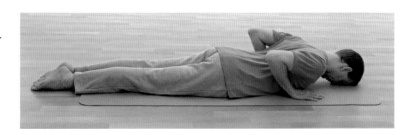

2 *As you inhale, lift both hands off the floor slightly. Then use the muscles of your neck and upper back to lift your head and chest. Hold your breath momentarily, then exhale and slowly lower your forehead and hands to the floor. Repeat the whole sequence 2 times. If you feel strong enough, you can hold the position for 3–5 breaths each time.*

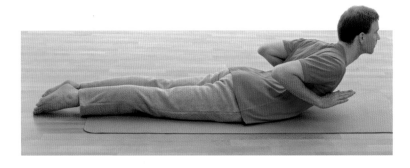

Full Basic Cobra

1 *Place your forehead on the mat and your hands next to your chest.*

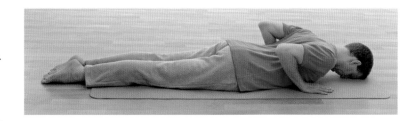

2 *As you inhale, slowly lift your chin, shoulders and chest off the floor, keeping your hips and hands grounded, and your elbows bent close in to your sides. As you exhale,*

slowly come back down, with your forehead being last to touch the mat. Repeat this 2 more times. With practice, you can hold this posture for up to 30 seconds.

3 *Once you are able to hold Step 2 for a number of breaths, try to lift the pose higher. Always make sure that it is the strength of the neck and upper back muscles that holds you in the position, rather than that of the arms. Again, hold this posture for up to 30 seconds, before exhaling and coming slowly back down to the floor, with your forehead being last to touch the mat.*

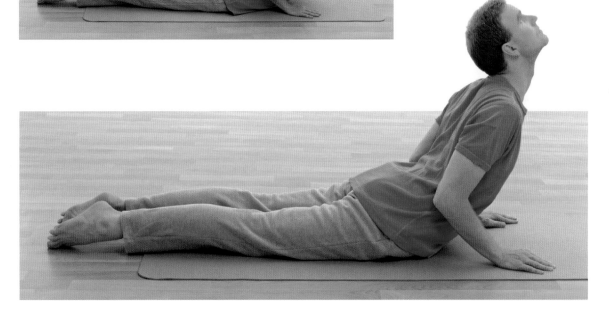

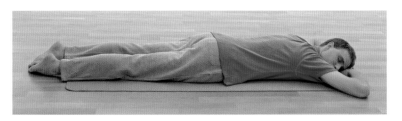

4 *Now just relax on the abdomen. Put one hand on top of the other, turn your head to one side and rest it there. Let the toes touch in the middle and drop the heels to each side. Be careful to keep the spine, neck and head in one line. Breathe slowly and rhythmically in the abdomen and relax the whole body.*

Cobra adaptation

If you experience any strain in the neck, resistance in the middle back or pain in the lower back while doing the posture, you may prefer to try the following variation.

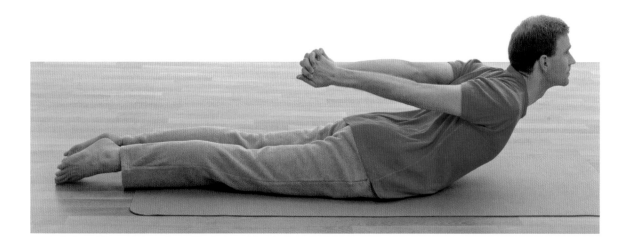

Lie on your front, stretch your arms behind your back and interlock your fingers. Then, as you inhale, slowly raise your head and chest, slightly lifting your hands and arms, and pulling them towards your feet. After a few deep breaths, slowly release the pose. This variation increases the flexibility of the shoulders and removes pressure from the lower back.

CHILD'S POSE ●

This soothing asana acts as a counter-pose to the backward bending exercises, and in particular the Cobra. It gently stretches the back muscles, releases pressure from the spine, brings more blood to the brain and gives the abdominal muscles a chance to relax. Once the body is in the position, no effort is required to hold the pose, which makes it ideal for deep relaxation.

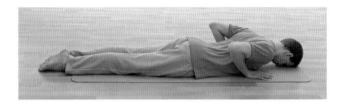

1 *Lie on your abdomen, rest your forehead on the floor and place your hands next to your chest.*

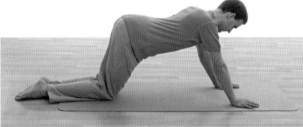

2 *As you inhale, push your hips up and come onto all fours.*

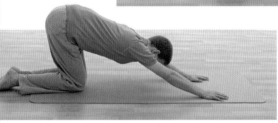

3 *As you exhale, stretch back like a cat, pushing your buttocks towards your heels, while stretching your arms on the floor in front of you.*

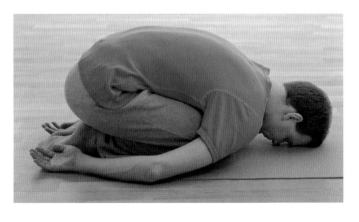

4 *Rest your buttocks on your heels if possible and place your forehead on the floor in front of your knees. Let your arms lie loosely alongside your legs, with your elbows slightly bent and relaxed. Remain here for 30–60 seconds.*

ALTERNATE NOSTRIL BREATHING ⦁▲

Anuloma viloma

Anuloma viloma, or Alternate Nostril Breathing, is the main form of *pranayama*, or breath regulation, presented in this book. Literally meaning 'control of prana', *pranayama* consists of specific breathing techniques that encourage the absorption of *prana* into the body's subtle energy channels (*nadis*) and energy centres (*chakras*), enhancing overall vitality and well-being.

Alternate Nostril Breathing corrects any negative breathing habits (see page 89), as well as helping you to balance how you use the two sides of your brain – the logical left side and the creative right side. Research has shown that there is a connection between this and the airflow in our nostrils: when the right nostril is more open, the left brain hemisphere is more active, and vice versa.

The Alternate Nostril Breathing exercise requires the use of two finger positions, known as *mudras* (see below), which help to focus the mind. The variations of this exercise offer different levels of *pranayama*, so start with the first one and only progress to the next once you feel entirely confident to do so.

The *mudras*

Two *mudras* are required for the practice of Alternate Nostril Breathing:

Vishnu mudra Lift your right arm, bend it at the elbow and bring your hand close to your nose. Then bend your index and middle fingers, gently pushing them against the palm of your hand to help move the mind towards inner concentration. During Alternate Nostril Breathing, you use your thumb to close the right nostril and your ring finger (the one beside your little one) to close the left nostril.

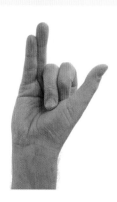

Chin mudra Place your left hand on your left knee, turning the palm upwards. Gently join the tip of the index finger (representing the individual consciousness) against the tip of the thumb (representing the cosmic consciousness). The other three fingers remain joined and extended in a relaxed position.

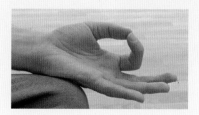

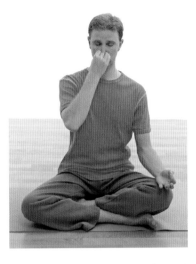
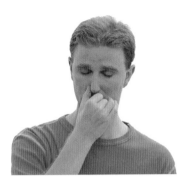
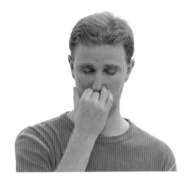

Variation 1: Single Nostril Breathing

1 *Sit in a cross-legged position, with your left hand in* chin mudra *(see left) on your left knee and your right hand in* vishnu mudra *(see left). Close your right nostril with your thumb and slowly exhale through the left nostril.*

2 *Inhale through your left nostril for 3 seconds, and exhale on the same side for 6 seconds. Repeat 3 more times.*

3 *Close your left nostril with your ring finger, release your thumb from your right nostril and inhale on the right side for 3 seconds, before exhaling on the same side for 6 seconds. Repeat 3 times. If you find this easy, try the next variation, otherwise continue with 3 more cycles of this exercise on each nostril.*

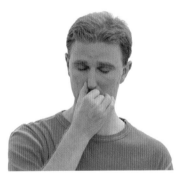
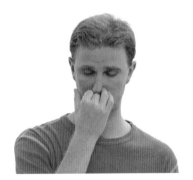

Variation 2: Alternate Breathing without Breath Retention

1 *Still cross-legged, close your right nostril with your thumb and release your left nostril to inhale on the left side for 3 seconds.*

2 *Then close your left nostril and release the right to exhale on the right side for 6 seconds. Then inhale on the right side for 3 seconds, switch nostrils again and exhale on the left side for 6 seconds. Repeat this whole* process 3 times to balance the brain hemispheres. If this practice is comfortable you may try the next variation. Otherwise practice up to 3 more rounds of this alternate breathing without retention.

THE LOCUST

Salabhasana

When the full version of this posture is practised (with both legs at a time), it resembles the jumping motion of a locust, hence the name. It provides excellent training for the lower back muscles, thus improving the quality of all sitting and standing activities. Plus, the full extension of the arms gives the arm muscles a healthy stretch. It is important with this posture always to do the Half Locust before progressing to the Full Locust.

Half Locust

1 *Lie on your abdomen, with your arms extended under your body, your hands clasped for stability (see inset picture) and your chin pointed forward on the mat.*

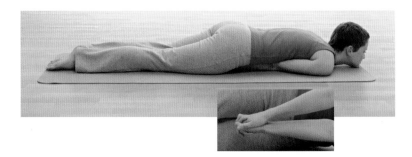

2 *As you inhale, slowly lift your right leg as high as possible behind you, keeping it straight and pointing your toes. Hold your breath for a few seconds as*

you remain in the pose, relaxing the left leg completely. As you exhale, slowly lower your right leg to the floor. Then repeat with your left leg. Practice this 4 more times on each side.

Relax on your abdomen, breathing deeply before progressing to the Full Locust if you feel comfortable to do so.

Full Locust

1 *Again, lie on your abdomen with your chin on the mat and extend both arms under your body, with hands either open or clasped.*

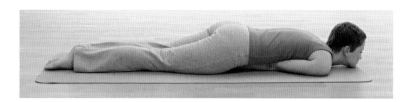

2 *Breathe in deeply and contract your back muscles. Lift both legs behind you, as high as you comfortably can, keeping them straight. It is more important to keep your legs completely straight than to get your legs up high. The main effort should be in your back muscles, helped by the contraction of your arm muscles. Hold your breath for a few seconds while you hold the pose. Then exhale and slowly lower your legs. Repeat 2 more times.*

Relax on your abdomen again, before entering Child's Pose (see page 83).

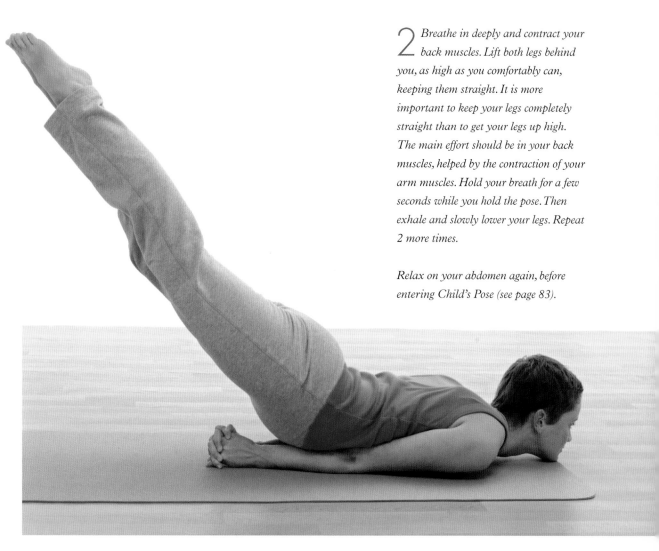

Class 4

Be aware that as your sessions become longer, you need to use more mental focus. This class introduces a wider range of movement to your yoga practice – the full Shoulderstand cycle (how to move smoothly from Shoulderstand into the Plough), a complete backbend (The Bow) and an introduction to Spinal Twist.

It also guides you in how to hold your breath for longer in Alternate Nostril Breathing (a form of *pranayama*), which will improve your physical and mental concentration. However, you should only attempt this if you already feel entirely comfortable with the breathing ratio suggested for Alternate Nostril Breathing in Class 3 (see pages 86–89).

How long does the class take?

10 minutes to read through the class
60–80 minutes to practise it for the first time
50–60 minutes when repeating the practice

Practice for busy people in 2 separate sessions (40–50 minutes):
Session A ●
Session B ▲

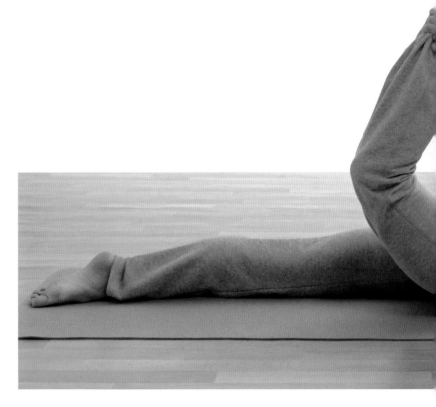

EXERCISE PLAN

✳ Indicates a new exercise

Initial Relaxation 2 minutes (pages 28–29) ● ▲
OM Chanting 3 times (page 30) ● ▲
Eye Exercises 5 times each (pages 31–33) ●
Relaxation Between Exercises (pages 46–47) ●
Neck Exercises 5 times each (pages 34–35) ▲
Relaxation Between Exercises (pages 46–47) ● ▲
✳ Alternate Nostril Breathing up to 6 rounds (page 94) ● ▲
Relaxation Between Exercises (pages 46–47) ● ▲
Sun Salutation 8 times (pages 64–71) ● ▲
Relaxation Between Exercises (pages 46–47) ● ▲
Single Leg Lifts 5 times each side (pages 42–45) ●
Relaxation Between Exercises (pages 46–47) ●
Double Leg Lifts 5 times (pages 48–49) ▲
Relaxation Between Exercises (pages 46–47) ▲
Shoulderstand 1–2 minutes (pages 50–51) ● ▲
✳ Shoulderstand to Plough 1 minute in total (page 95) ● ▲
Relaxation Between Exercises (pages 46–47) ● ▲
The Fish 1 minute (pages 74–75) ● ▲
Relaxation Between Exercises (pages 46–47) ● ▲
Forward Bend 1–2 minutes (pages 76–78) ●
Inclined Plane 30 seconds (page 79) ●

Relaxation Between Exercises (pages 46–47) ●
The Cobra 30 seconds (pages 80–82) ▲
Relaxation on the abdomen 1 minute (Step 4, page 81) ▲
Half Locust 5 times (page 90) ▲
Relaxation on the abdomen 1 minute (Step 4, page 81) ▲
Full Locust 3 times (page 91) ▲
Relaxation on the abdomen 1 minute (Step 4, page 81) ▲
✳ The Bow 3 times (pages 96–97) ●
Relaxation on the abdomen 1 minute (Step 4, page 81) ●
Child's Pose 30 seconds (page 83) ● ▲
✳ Half Spinal Twist up to 1 minute each side (pages 98–101) ▲
Child's Pose 30 seconds (page 83) ▲
Final Relaxation 10–15 minutes (pages 54–57) ● ▲

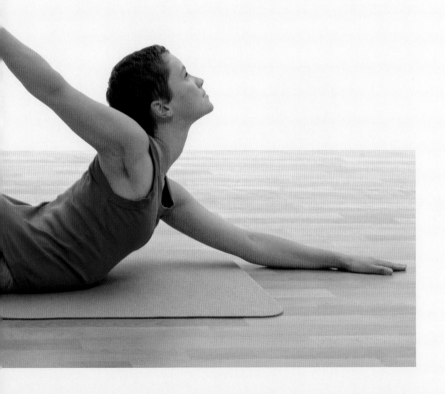

ALTERNATE NOSTRIL BREATHING ⁝

Anuloma viloma

This breathing exercise is an extension of Variation 3 of *anuloma viloma* on pages 86–89 and should only be attempted once you feel completely comfortable with that, which has a breath ratio of 3:6:6 (inhaling:holding:exhaling). The breath will now be held for twice as long now, as the ratio is 3:12:6.

This extended breath retention gently stimulates the heart and allows the nervous system to relax more deeply, as well as increasing energy circulation. If you still find Variation 3 on page 88 difficult, continue developing it before trying this one.

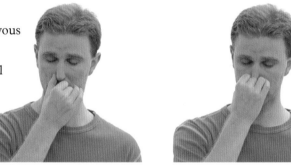

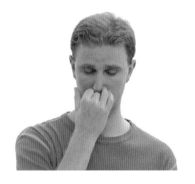

1 *Sitting cross-legged, close your right nostril with your right thumb and inhale on the left side for 3 seconds.*

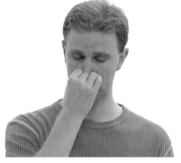

2 *Then use your ring finger to close the other nostril too and hold your breath for 12 seconds.*

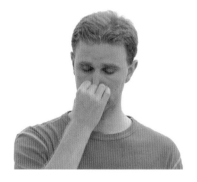

3 *Release your thumb to exhale on the right side for 6 seconds. Then inhale on the same side for 3 seconds.*

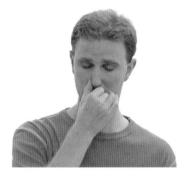

4 *Close both nostrils again and hold your breath for 12 seconds.*

5 *Release your ring finger to exhale on the left side for 6 seconds. Practise Steps 1–5 up to 6 times.*

Then rest and relax on your back in Corpse Pose for 1–2 minutes (see pages 46–47).

SHOULDERSTAND TO PLOUGH

Sarvangasana to Halasana

Learning to move smoothly between Shoulderstand and the Plough, without any relaxation between them as in previous classes, further builds strength in the lower back muscles, which is very important for all standing and sitting positions in daily life. This transition also improves the harmonious flow of your yoga practice. The guidance here starts in Shoulderstand position as this has been covered already on pages 50–53.

1 Make sure that your spine is as vertical as possible and that you are firmly supporting your back with both hands while in Shoulderstand posture. After holding the asana for 1–2 minutes, start to move into the Plough position by slowly lowering your legs behind your head towards the floor, supporting your back with both hands and flexing the toes (see also pages 72–73).

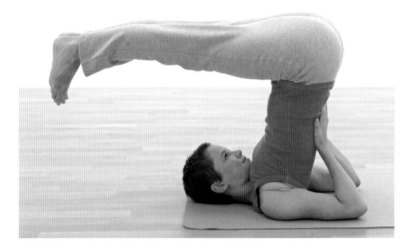

2 If your feet touch the ground, lower your arms to the floor behind your back. If your feet do not touch the floor yet, keep supporting the back with both hands for stability. Hold this position for up to 1 minute. Then support your back again with both hands, inhale, lift both legs back up to Shoulderstand and slowly release your legs to the floor.

Relax in Corpse Pose for about 1 minute (see pages 46–47) before moving on to the next posture.

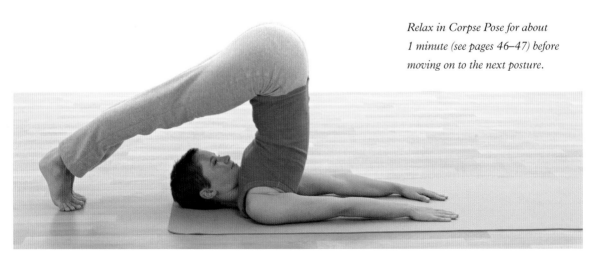

HALF SPINAL TWIST ▲

Ardha Matsyendrasana

The position of the arms and legs in Half Spinal Twist may look
a little complicated at first, but with practice you will discover that
it is actually a very simple and intelligent way to progressively
improve your body's ability for rotational movement. The twist
keeps the spine elastic, tones the spinal nerve roots and the
sympathetic nervous system, and alleviates constipation by
applying pressure to the large intestine.

Spinal Twist Preparations

These exercises below serve as a progressive introduction to Half
Spinal Twist. You may need to practise them for a few weeks until
the hips are flexible enough to do Half Spinal Twist itself. Once
you can manage Half Spinal Twist, however, there is no need to do
these warm-ups every time.

PREPARATION 1

*Kneel on your mat, with your spine
upright, and sit on your heels. Turn
your head to the left and start twisting
by moving your left arm behind you
until your hand is on the floor behind
your back, as far towards the right side
of your body as you can reach. At the
same time, place your right hand on
the outside of your left knee and apply
a little pressure here to increase the
rotation of the thoracic vertebrae.
Breathe deeply and rhythmically.
Then slowly release the pose and
practise the rotation to the other side.*

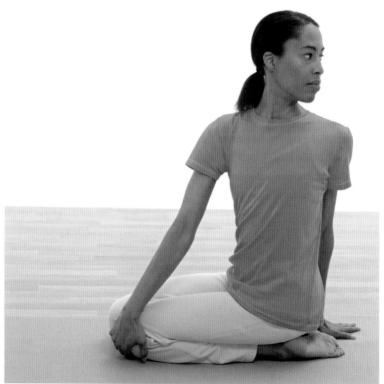

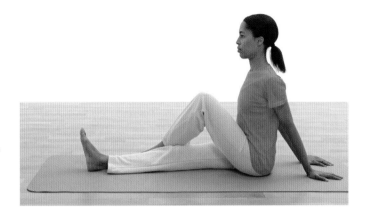

PREPARATION 2

1 Sit with both legs extended in front of you. Bend your left leg, placing the left foot on the floor, just outside your right calf.

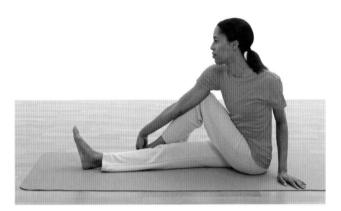

2 Bring your right arm around the outside of your left leg and catch hold of either your calf, ankle or foot, depending on your flexibility.

3 Keeping your spine upright, continue twisting by moving your left arm behind you until your hand is on the floor behind your back, as far towards the right side of your body as *you can reach. Look over your left shoulder, without straining your neck. Hold the pose for 30 seconds. Then slowly release the pose and practise the rotation to the other side.*

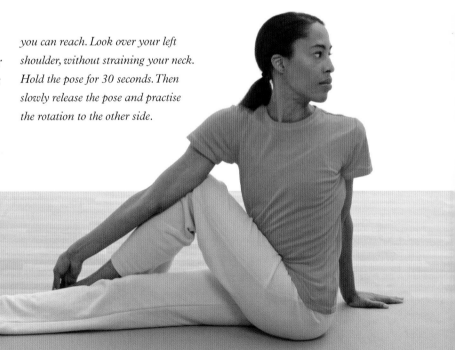

Class 5

By now you will be quite familiar with the key elements of yoga practice: asanas, breathing and relaxation. In the previous classes, you have mostly practised breathing and relaxation techniques separately from postures. In this class, the challenge is now to remain aware of your breathing and relaxation while you are moving into and holding each pose. A further extension of Alternate Nostril Breathing is also provided, teaching you, yet again, to breathe in a more balanced, controlled way, thus further enhancing your powers of concentration. Two new standing poses – Standing Forward Bend and the Triangle – are also introduced at the end of the class to provide additional strength and flexibility for the whole body.

How long does the class take?

10 minutes to read through the class
75–90 minutes to practise it for the first time
60–75 minutes when repeating the practice

Practice for busy people in 2 separate sessions (50–60 minutes):
Session A ●
Session B ▲

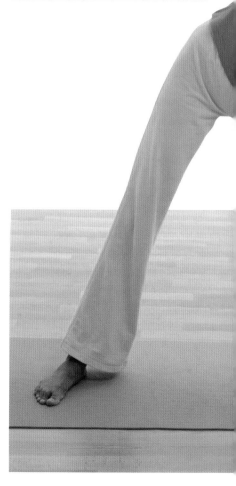

EXERCISE PLAN

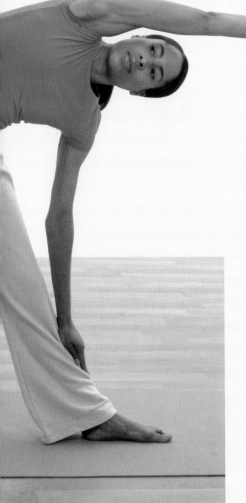

✳ Indicates a new exercise

ALTERNATE NOSTRIL BREATHING

Anuloma viloma

If you are comfortable with the practice of Alternate Nostril Breathing for the count of 3:12:6 on page 94, you can try to increase the count slightly with this exercise. Otherwise, simply continue the variation on page 94 or a previous, less challenging variation if appropriate (see pages 86–89).

The extended breathing ratio here further stimulates the heart and deepens relaxation. Be careful when trying this new exercise, however, as the increase of the breathing ratio in any *pranayama* must be done very gradually. If you move up to a higher count too quickly, the stimulating effect can be too strong, which will result in a wave of tension in the nervous system – the very opposite of the desired energy control.

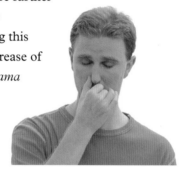

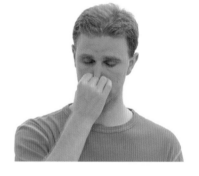

1 *Sitting cross-legged, close your right nostril with your right thumb and inhale on the left side for 4 seconds.*

2 *Then use your ring finger to close the other nostril too and hold your breath for 16 seconds.*

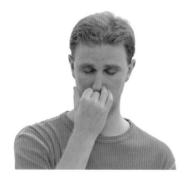

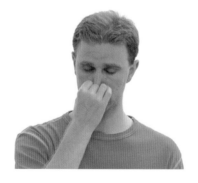

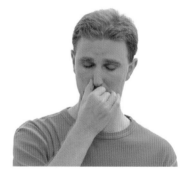

3 *Release your thumb to exhale on the right side for 8 seconds. Then inhale on the same side for 4 seconds.*

4 *Close both nostrils again and hold your breath for 16 seconds.*

5 *Release your ring finger to exhale on the left side for 8 seconds. Practise Steps 1–5 6 times in all.*

Then rest and relax on your back for 1 minute (see pages 46–47).

STANDING FORWARD BEND •

Pada hastasana

This posture, whose Sanskrit name literally means 'Hand to Foot Pose' – is a natural continuation of the sitting Forward Bend on pages 76–78. This time, a greater stretch is achieved due to the larger range of movement, stretching the hamstrings, making the spine more supple and increasing blood circulation in the head.

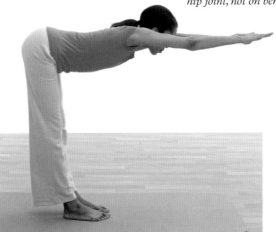

1 *Stand with your feet about 5 cm (2 in) apart, inhale and lift your arms in the air, next to your ears.*

2 *Exhale and bend forward from your hips, keeping your legs straight and your body as extended as possible. Progress in the forward bend depends on the quality of the angle you create at the hip joint, not on bending the spine itself.*

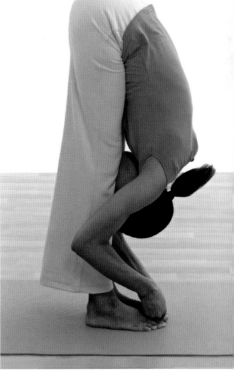

3 *Aim to hook your big toes with your index fingers (the classical foot-hold; see page 77). If this is not possible, then catch hold of your ankles or calves with your hands. Only bend down as far as is possible with straight legs. Keeping your shoulders relaxed, use the pull of gravity to gradually increase the*

forward bend with each breath. Hold the pose for up to 1 minute and then slowly curl up to standing position, keeping your arms and hands hanging loose as you do so.

Take a few deep breaths in standing position before continuing with the next pose.

THE TRIANGLE ▲

Trikonasana

The Triangle posture entails lateral, or sideways, bending, which completes the range of spinal movement in the asana session. In this position, lateral bending occurs mainly in the lumbar (lower), as well as in the thoracic (central) area. The Triangle is a very active pose that places equal emphasis on stretching, strengthening and balancing. It simultaneously stretches, contracts and relaxes all the major back muscles, increasing spinal flexibility as well as providing the abdominal organs with a stimulating massage.

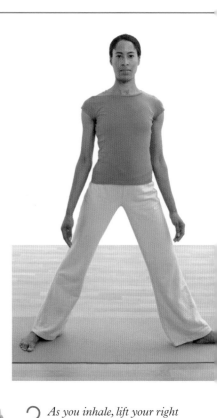

1 *Stand with your legs about double shoulder-width apart and turn your left foot 90 degrees to the left. Breathe rhythmically into your abdomen and distribute your weight evenly on both feet.*

2 *Lift both arms out wide, at shoulder height.*

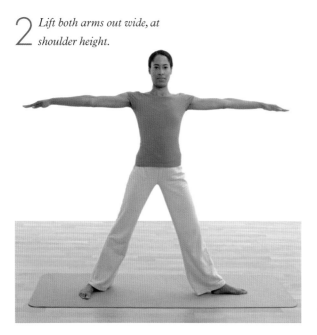

3 *As you inhale, lift your right arm up towards your right ear, palm facing inwards. Keep your left arm out to the side at shoulder height.*

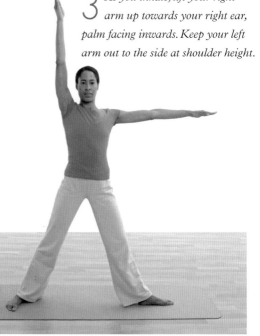

4 *As you slowly exhale, bend to your left side, until your right arm is over your head and parallel to the floor and your left hand is reaching down to your left ankle. Keep your right arm against your right ear, and turn your gaze upwards. Hold the pose for between 15 and 30 seconds, breathing deeply. As you inhale, reach back up to standing position, then exhale and release your right arm. If you need to, shake out your legs, then repeat the exercise, bending laterally to your right side. Repeat 2 times on each side.*

Then proceed to Final Relaxation (see pages 54–57).

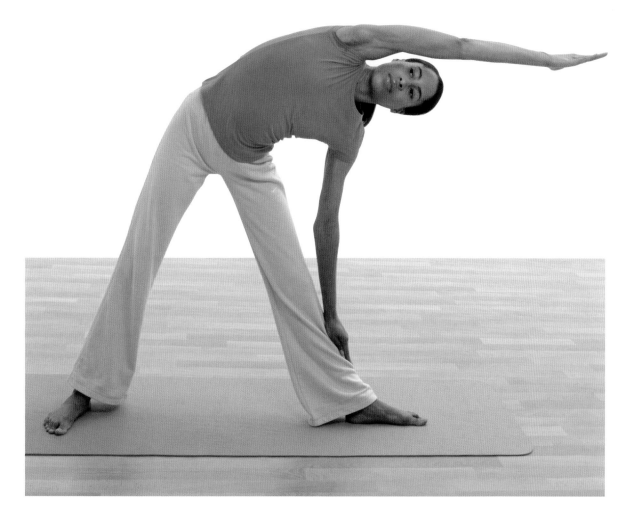

Class 6

Welcome to Class 6. Having progressed through the yoga classes until this stage, you have now learned almost all 12 basic yoga postures, as well as all the main tools for doing them mindfully and effectively. By this stage, you are likely to have noticed that yoga improves your general sensory coordination, not only during yoga exercises but also in daily life. You are likely to find yourself doings all sorts of tasks with more ease, from walking to climbing a ladder to being able to work more efficiently.

This class introduces a new, vigorous breathing exercise that teaches you how to purify your lungs by completely emptying them in a series of strong exhalations. At the same time, the inhalations are completely relaxed, which recharges energy levels. This class also guides you through a movement known as the Dolphin, which prepares you for the only one of the 12 basic postures that you have not yet experienced – Headstand.

The class then ends with a systematic training of your sense of balance, offering you a choice between three balancing poses: the relatively easy Tree posture, the more challenging Crow and the more advanced Peacock.

How long does the class take?

10 minutes to read through the class
75–90 minutes to practise it for the first time
60–75 minutes when repeating the practice

Practice for busy people in 2 separate sessions (50–60 minutes):
Session A ●
Session B ▲

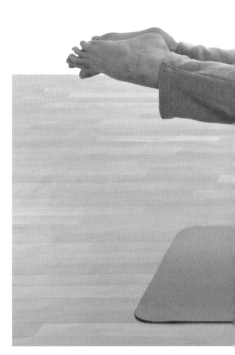

EXERCISE PLAN

❋ Indicates a new exercise

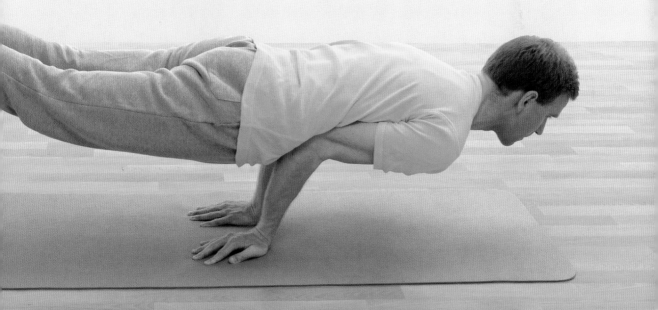

LUNG PURIFICATION

Kapala bhati

The active exhalations in *kapala bhati* help to empty the lungs to their maximum, developing their vital capacity; the rhythmical contractions of the abdomen increase the return of blood from the abdomen to the heart, increasing the strength of the heartbeat; and all abdominal organs are stimulated. The increased breath retention also allows accumulation of *prana*, leading to increased powers of concentration. Plus, *kapala bhati* can help to overcome smoking. However, this exercise should never be practised shortly before going to bed, as its stimulating effect may prevent sleep.

Learning passive inhalation

When we contract the abdomen, our diaphragm pushes air out. However, no effort is necessarily required to bring air back into the lungs: we can automatically or passively breathe in when we simply relax the abdomen after the contraction. The exercise below will get you used to doing this so that you can put it into practice during the actual Lung Purification exercise.

Caution

When practising *kapala bhati* for the first time, dizziness or hyperventilation may occur if you do it incorrectly, so make sure only the abdomen is moving, both in inhalation and exhalation (not the chest or collar bone). At the least sign of dizziness, immediately stop the practice, lie down and relax on your back.

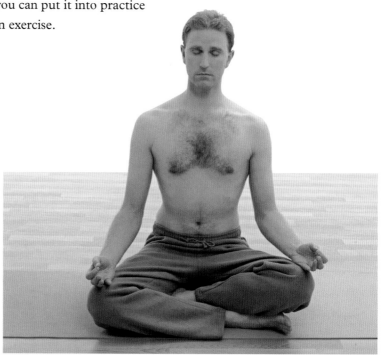

Preparation

Sitting cross-legged, actively inhale, allowing your abdomen to expand. Then slowly exhale and continue contracting your abdomen until your lungs are emptied to the maximum. Hold the contraction for a moment, then suddenly and completely relax your abdomen. You will feel how the air automatically enters into your lungs. Repeat this a number of times until you feel more comfortable with it.

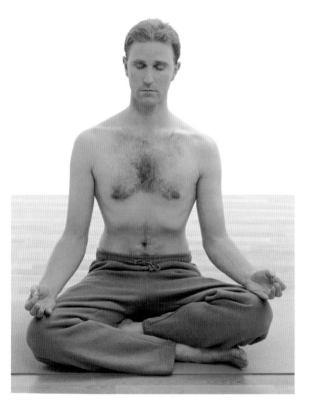 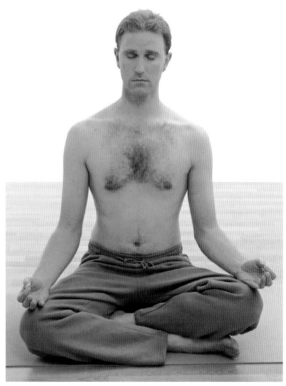

Lung Purification

1 *Sit cross-legged, with both hands on your knees in* chin mudra *(see page 86). After a comfortable abdominal inhalation, rhythmically contract and relax your abdomen 20 times in order to exhale and inhale 20 times in a row through your nose. Each active exhalation should be as short and energetic as possible and each passive inhalation should take about 1 second. Make sure that when your abdomen comes in, the air is actually pushed out, and that the inhalation is noiseless and effortless.*

2 *After the last forceful exhalation, take two slow Complete Yogic Breaths (see pages 60–63), followed by a comfortable inhalation. Then, with your eyes closed, hold your breath for 20–60 seconds, according to your capacity. Then slowly exhale. Practise 2 more rounds.*

Finally, rest for 1–2 minutes in Relaxation Pose on your back (see pages 46–47).

THE CROW ▲

Kakasana

The asanas to date have focused mainly on strength and flexibility of the spine. The Crow posture, however, as well as the Tree and the Peacock, are balancing poses. Although the Crow may look difficult at first, it is important to bear in mind that all the previous breathing exercises and postures actually prepare for balancing: controlled breathing allows you to focus your energies on a balancing point and the asanas have trained your body to fine-tune the contraction and relaxation of muscles.

As well as increasing your sense of balance, the Crow greatly strengthens the wrists and arms. If it is too difficult at first, try the Tree instead – a variant balancing pose. And once you are comfortable with both the Tree and the Crow, you can progress to the more challenging Peacock pose. Bear in mind, though, that one balancing pose per yoga session is enough.

1 *Squat with your feet slightly apart, your knees bent and your hands placed on the mat in front of you.*

2 *Keeping your hands flat on the floor and your fingers spread out, bend your upper arms slightly out to the side, under your knees. Keep your forearms apart, at an angle of approximately 90 degrees, creating a small platform just on top of your elbows where your knees can be placed.*

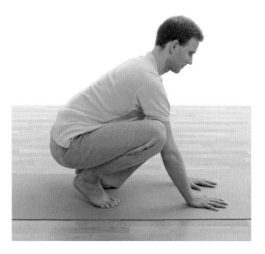

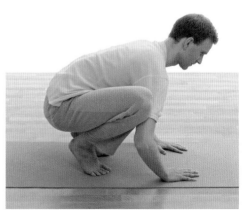

3 *Lift up onto your toes, look up slightly and slowly lean forward, bringing more weight onto your hands and arms.*

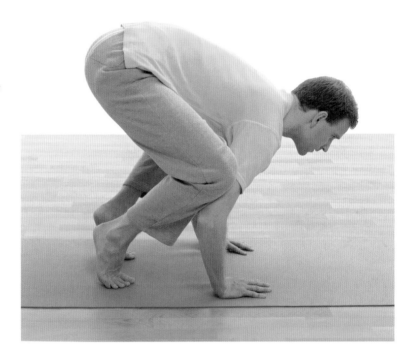

4 *Inhale deeply and, if you feel comfortable to do so, continue to lean forward until your feet come off the floor and you are left balancing on your hands. Breathe slowly and rhythmically, concentrating on a spot in the wall in front of you or on the horizon for balance.*

Then move back onto your feet and rest and relax in Child's Pose (see page 83).

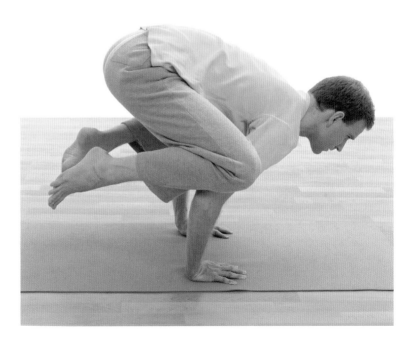

Class 7

This class introduces only one new exercise – Half Headstand – in the lead-up to teaching you the last of the 12 basic postures - Full Headstand – in Class 8. In yoga, Headstand is considered to be the 'king of asanas' due to the remarkable benefits it brings to brain power, memory and concentration. Learning to balance upside down can bring you great confidence, but be sure to practise it carefully, only after you have studied all the information about the technique and contraindications.

Like the classes before it, this asana session covers all five basic principles of yoga: the asanas mobilize the spine and all the joints ('proper exercise'); breathing exercises circulate the vital energy ('proper breathing'); relaxation techniques release tensions ('proper relaxation'); increased circulation brings nutrients to and removes waste materials from all the body's cells ('proper diet'). The alternating pattern of exercise and relaxation enhances positive thinking, and the concentration required to incorporate all these aspects can bring about a meditative state ('positive thinking and meditation').

How long does the class take?

10 minutes to read through the class
75–90 minutes to practise it for the first time
60–75 minutes when repeating the practice

Practice for busy people in 2 separate sessions (50–60 minutes):
Session A ●
Session B ▲

EXERCISE PLAN

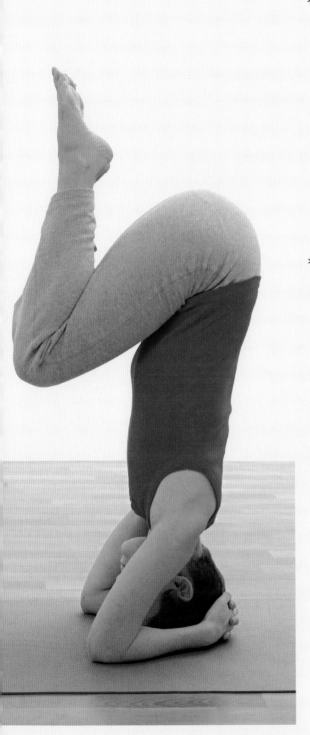

✳ Indicates a new exercise

Initial Relaxation 2 minutes (pages 28–29) ● ▲
OM Chanting 3 times (page 30) ● ▲
Eye Exercises (optional) (pages 31–33)
Relaxation Between Exercises (optional) (pages 46–47)
Neck Exercises (optional) (pages 34–35)
Relaxation Between Exercises (optional) (pages 46–47)
Lung Purification 3 rounds of 30 exhalations (pages 110–111) ●
Alternate Nostril Breathing 3 6 rounds of 4:16:8 (page 104) ▲
Relaxation Between Exercises (pages 46–47) ▲
Sun Salutation 10 times (pages 64–71) ● ▲
Relaxation Between Exercises (pages 46–47) ● ▲
Single Leg Lifts 5 times each side (pages 42–45) ●
Double Leg Lifts 5 times (pages 48–49) ▲
Relaxation Between Exercises (pages 46–47) ▲
The Dolphin up to 10 times (pages 112–113) ● ▲
Child's Pose 30 seconds (see page 83) ● ▲
✳ Half Headstand up to 1 minute (pages 120–123) ● ▲
Child's Pose 30 seconds (page 83) ● ▲
Relaxation Between Exercises (pages 46–47) ● ▲
Shoulderstand 1–2 minutes (Steps 1–3, pages 50–53) ● ▲
The Plough 1 minute (Steps 4–5, pages 72–73) ▲
Relaxation Between Exercises (pages 46–47) ● ▲
The Fish 1 minute (pages 74–75) ● ▲
Relaxation Between Exercises (pages 46–47) ● ▲
Forward Bend 1–2 minutes (pages 76–78) ●
Inclined Plane 30 seconds (page 79) ●
Relaxation Between Exercises (pages 46–47) ●
The Cobra 30 seconds (pages 80–82) ▲
Relaxation on the abdomen 1 minute (Step 4, page 81) ▲
Half Locust 30 seconds (page 90) ▲
Relaxation on the abdomen 30 seconds (Step 4, page 81) ▲
Full Locust 30 seconds (page 91) ▲
Relaxation on the abdomen 30 seconds (Step 4, page 81) ▲
The Bow 2 x 30 seconds (pages 96–97) ●
Relaxation on the abdomen 1 minute (Step 4, page 81) ●
Child's Pose 1 minute (page 83) ●
Half Spinal Twist 1 minute each side (pages 98–101) ●
Child's Pose 30 seconds (page 83) ●
The Crow/Tree/Peacock 30 seconds (pages 114–117) ▲
Child's Pose 30 seconds (page 83) ▲
Standing Forward Bend 1 minute (pages 104–105) ●
The Triangle 30 seconds each side (pages 106–107) ▲
Final Relaxation 10–15 minutes (pages 54–57) ● ▲

HALF HEADSTAND ⚇

Sirshasana preparation

The headstand is a boon for developing brain power and a healthy heart, and the beauty of it is that absolutely anyone of any age can do it. To the surprise of many people, it does not require any special strength or flexibility; all you need to do is respect certain basic considerations and follow the step-by-step guidelines given. Once you have learned it, it feels as natural to stand on your head as to stand on your feet.

You may wonder how the small vertebrae of the cervical region can support the weight of the body, which in the upright position is carried by the large vertebrae of the lumbar area. The answer is that they do not have to: during Headstand, more than half of the body weight should actually be placed on the arms. The remaining weight can be taken by the head, as long as the neck is properly aligned with the rest of the spinal column. When doing the exercise below, you may wish to place a blanket and some pillows on the mat behind you, in case you accidentally roll over while attempting it.

Caution

Do not do Headstand if you suffer from high blood pressure, glaucoma, a detached retina, any infections affecting your head (from ear infections to head colds), any neck injury, or during menstruation and pregnancy. If you have any doubts regarding these contraindications, make sure you consult with your doctor before attempting Headstand. If you have any postural or alignment problems, you may only be able to hold Headstand for a short time. Always release the pose as soon as you feel any discomfort in the neck area.

1 Kneel on your mat, lean forward, place each hand around the opposite elbow and lean your arms on the floor. The distance between your elbows should correspond approximately to the breadth of your shoulders.

2 Keeping your elbows where they are, move your hands forward and interlock your fingers. This creates a firm triangular base with your elbows and hands, with equal weight on all three points of the triangle. Mentally affirm: 'My arms are my legs' to help you to keep the maximum amount of weight on this 'tripod'.

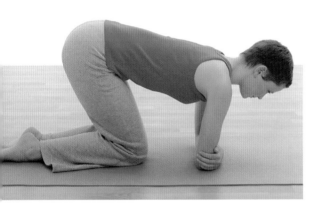

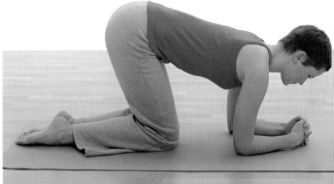

3 Place the top of your head on the mat, with your hands firmly supporting the back of your head.

4 Lift up onto your toes, with your hips in the air and your legs straight. Continue to press your elbows and hands firmly against the mat.

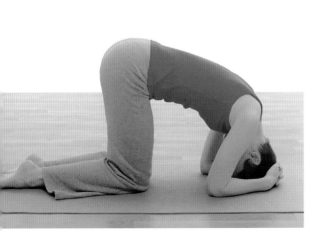

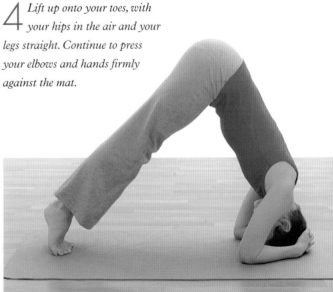

5 With straight legs, walk your feet in towards your head, until your back is as vertical as possible. Keep pressing the weight on the supporting tripod you have made with your arms. Then either lower your knees to the floor and relax in Child's Pose for a few breaths (see page 83) or move on to Step 6. Do not, however, progress to Step 6 until you are completely comfortable with Steps 1–5. Remember, it does not matter how long this takes you. There is no rush.

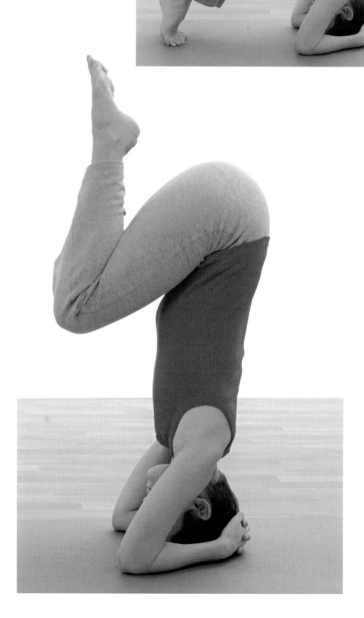

6 When you feel ready to progress, bend your legs and slowly lift your feet off the floor. Do not try to 'jump' or 'kick up' and do not try to straighten your legs as you could easily lose balance doing this and fall straight on your back. Instead, slowly tilt your pelvis backwards until you find the point of balance in your lower back. In this position, the weight of your bent legs is balanced by the weight of your hips and buttocks. Keep as much support as possible on your forearms and hands, breathe rhythmically and hold the asana for up to 1 minute. Then come down very gradually in the opposite order you went up in – bringing your feet to the floor first, walking them away from the body and then bringing your knees slowly to the floor.

Remain in Child's Pose for a few moments (see page 83), then rest and relax on your back (see pages 46–47).

Assessing your progress

If you are unable to lift your feet and back up into Half
Headstand in Step 6, it is most likely due to a lack of flexibility
in your hamstrings and lower back muscles, which prevents
you from walking close enough to your head in Step 5. You
can gauge how easily you will be able to come up into Half
Headstand by observing your flexibility in the Forward Bend
(see pages 76–78):

If your Forward Bend is limited (see below), you are
unlikely to be able to walk your feet far enough
towards your head in Step 5 (see opposite) to be able
to rise in a slow, controlled manner into the posture. In
this case, you should only practise this exercise with an
experienced teacher who will be able to help you
safely into Step 6 of Half Headstand.

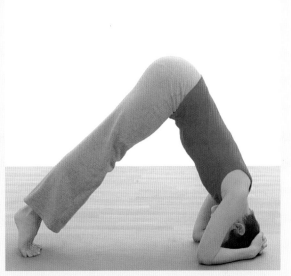

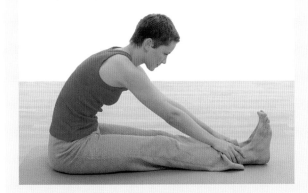

If you practise the Forward Bend (see below), you will
gradually improve the flexibility of your lower back
and hamstrings. This will enable you to get your spine
vertical and your feet closer to your head in Step 5
(see opposite) – allowing you to move into Half
Headstand with both legs at a time.

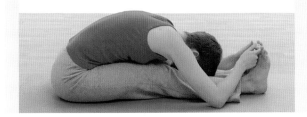

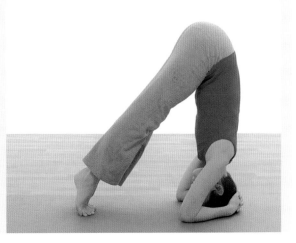

Class 8

Congratulations! You are about to practise the complete yoga programme. Out of hundreds of classical yoga exercises, this session of 12 basic asanas, with counter-poses, warm-ups, breathing exercises and deep relaxation was developed by the great yoga masters of the Himalayas.

Swami Vishnu-devananda first introduced this practice to the West in 1957, and since then several generations of yoga students, from all over the world, have made it an integral part of their lives.

The combined benefits of this practice sequence in the order given are far superior to the effects of any of the single exercises. The breathing exercises (*pranayamas*) oxygenate all the body's cells and gently increase the circulation. Sun Salutation stretches and warms up almost all the body's muscles. The 12 basic asanas, including full Headstand posture, systematically improve muscle length and strength, mobilize the joints and move the spine in all possible directions. The asanas apply pressure to various parts of the body, massaging the internal organs and releasing *prana* in the energy channels (*nadis*) and energy centres (*chakras*). And Final Relaxation provides complete rest for all the body's systems and for the mind, as well as connecting us to the inner spiritual strength of the Soul.

How long does the class take?

10 minutes to read through the class
75–90 minutes to practise it for the first time
60–75 minutes when repeating the practice

Practice for busy people in 2 separate sessions (50–60 minutes):
Session A ●
Session B ▲

Do not worry if you do not feel ready to do the full Headstand posture yet; you can simply continue to do Half Headstand (see pages 120–123) until you feel confident. You should always do every posture at a level that is comfortable for you on any given day because your body will react differently at different times. This means it is fine to revert to easier options and progressions in earlier classes when necessary. This might be the case if you miss a few sessions or if your yoga practice has been slightly sporadic of late, or you may be able to do a full Class 8 but at a more gentle rate. In case of long-term interruption, however, you should start again with Class 1 and continue, class by class.

EXERCISE PLAN

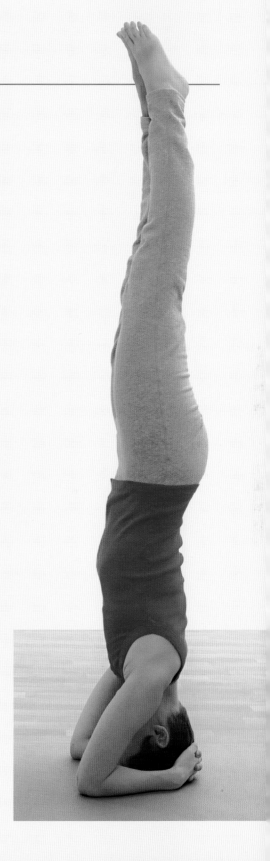

✳ Indicates a new exercise

Initial Relaxation 2 minutes (pages 28–29) ● ▲
OM Chanting 3 times (page 30) ● ▲
Eye Exercises (optional) (pages 31–33)
Relaxation Between Exercises (optional) (pages 46–47)
Neck Exercises (optional) (pages 34–35)
Relaxation Between Exercises (optional) (pages 46–47)
Lung Purification 3 rounds of 40 exhalations (pages 110–111) ●
Relaxation Between Exercises (pages 46–47) ●
Alternate Nostril Breathing 6 rounds of 4:16:8 (page 104) ▲
Relaxation Between Exercises 1 minute (pages 46–47) ▲
Sun Salutation 10 times (pages 64–71) ● ▲
Relaxation Between Exercises 1 minute (pages 46–47) ● ▲
Single Leg Lifts 5 times each side (pages 42–45) ●
Double Leg Lifts 5 times (pages 48–49) ▲
Relaxation Between Exercises 1 minute (pages 46–47) ▲
The Dolphin 5 to 10 times (pages 112–113) ●
Child's Pose 30 seconds (page 83) ●
Half Headstand up to 1 minute (pages 120–123) ● ▲
✳ Headstand 2 x 30–60 seconds (pages 126–127) ● ▲
Child's Pose 30 seconds (page 83) ● ▲
Relaxation Between Exercises 1 minute (pages 46–47) ● ▲
Shoulderstand 1–2 minutes (Steps 1–3, pages 50–53) ● ▲
The Plough 1 minute (Steps 4–5, pages 72–73) ▲
Relaxation Between Exercises 1 minute (pages 46–47) ● ▲
The Fish 1 minute (pages 74–75) ● ▲
Relaxation Between Exercises 1 minute (pages 46–47) ● ▲
Forward Bend 1–2 minutes (pages 76–78) ●
Inclined Plane 30 seconds (page 79) ●
Relaxation Between Exercises 1 minute (pages 46–47) ●
The Cobra 30 seconds (pages 80–82) ▲
Relaxation on the abdomen 1 minute (Step 4, page 81) ▲
Half Locust 30 seconds (page 90) ▲
Relaxation on the abdomen 30 seconds (Step 4, page 81) ▲
Full Locust 30 seconds (page 91) ▲
Relaxation on the abdomen 30 seconds (Step 4, page 81) ▲
The Bow 2 x 30 seconds (pages 96–97) ●
Relaxation on the abdomen 1 minute (Step 4, page 81) ●
Child's Pose 1 minute (page 83) ●
Half Spinal Twist 1 minute each side (pages 98–101) ●
Child's Pose 30 seconds (page 83) ●
The Crow/Tree/Peacock 30 seconds (pages 114–117) ▲
Child's Pose 30 seconds (page 83) ▲
Standing Forward Bend 1 minute (pages 104–105) ●
The Triangle 30 seconds each side (pages 106–107) ▲
Final Relaxation 10–15 minutes (pages 54–57) ● ▲

HEADSTAND

Sirshasana

Day in day out, our brain enables our body to carry out all its voluntary and involuntary functions. Headstand provides us with the perfect opportunity to give something back to our poor, overworked and under-rewarded brain. During this inverted posture, the body sends a rich supply of oxygenated blood to the brain, greatly enhancing memory and concentration. For this reason the headstand is considered the 'king of asanas'. It also strengthens the heartbeat due to increased venous return to the heart and relieves any pressure on the lower back.

Once you are able to balance the body safely in Step 6 of Half Headstand (see page 122) you can try the complete Headstand position below. Many people, however, will only learn the full Headstand with the help of a qualified and competent teacher.

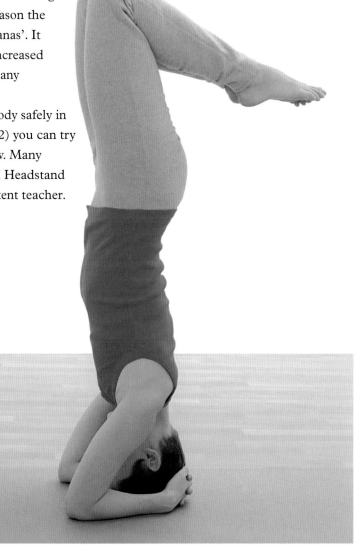

1 *Keeping your hips firmly in place in Half Headstand position from page 122, slowly lift your knees until they point upwards. Focus on the balance in your lower back, so that your body neither topples forwards or backwards. Maintain the weight on the tripod of your arms and hands as much as possible. Breathe rhythmically, keep your knees bent and be careful not to let your back arch.*

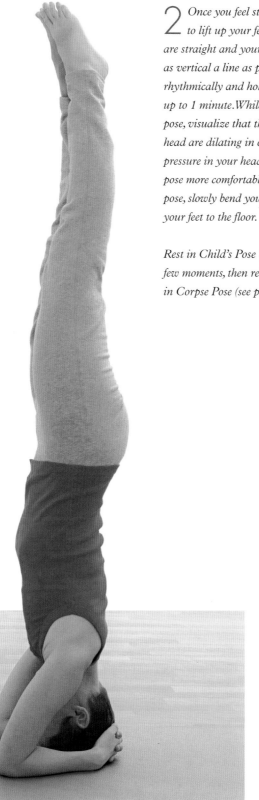

2 *Once you feel steady, slowly start to lift up your feet until your legs are straight and your whole body is in as vertical a line as possible. Breathe rhythmically and hold the asana for up to 1 minute. While holding the pose, visualize that the arteries in your head are dilating in order to reduce pressure in your head and to make the pose more comfortable. To release the pose, slowly bend your knees and lower your feet to the floor.*

Rest in Child's Pose (see page 83) for a few moments, then relax on your back in Corpse Pose (see pages 46–47).

Why you should not practise Headstand against a wall

There are a number of very good reasons not to learn Headstand against a wall:

• When your feet touch the wall, your attention is drawn from your hands and arms to your feet and legs. This would increase the weight on your head and could be harmful to your neck.

• Bringing your feet towards the wall would exaggerate the curve in your lower back and therefore prevent correct alignment.

• If you fall over, your neck could easily become twisted, with the rest of your body collapsing on top of it.

• Practising against a wall becomes a habit that means you might become too frightened to practise without a wall after a certain period

CHAPTER 2

Nutrition

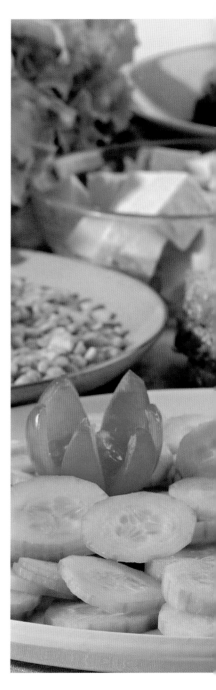

'The Yogi considers, using both his knowledge of nutrition and his internal experience, which foods can be consumed in what minimum quantity with the most positive effect on the body and the mind, and with the least negative impact on the environment and least pain to other beings.'
Swami Vishnu-devananda

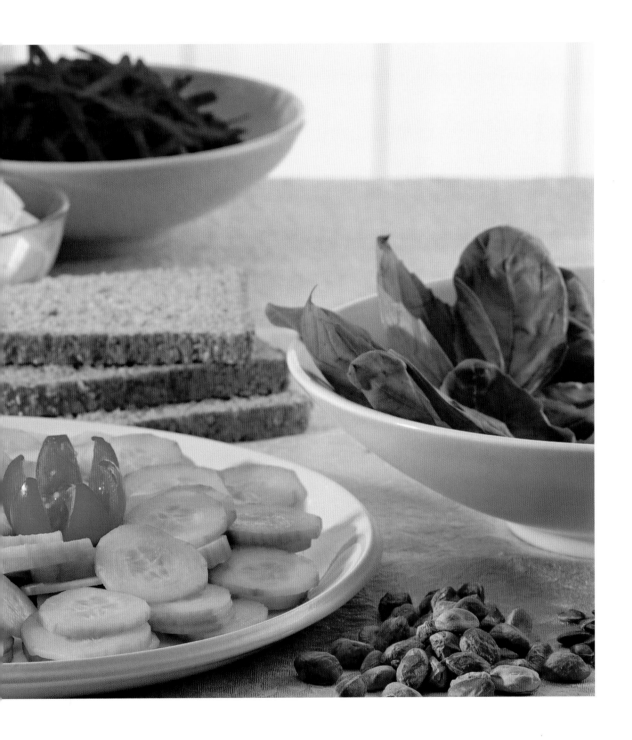

BENEFITS OF VEGETARIANISM

Yogic tradition advocates a lacto-vegetarian diet: avoiding the consumption of fish, eggs and meat (both red and white), and limiting your intake of dairy products. The main motivation for this is a heightened sensitivity to the taking of innocent animal life and to the cruel conditions of industrial animal farming and dairy production. This non-violent approach is known, in yogic terms, as *ahimsa*. A well-balanced vegetarian diet has been proven to be extremely healthy and highly preventive against many of today's most common degenerative diseases.

High blood pressure, arteriosclerosis (hardening of the arteries due to plaque deposits on the walls of the blood vessels) and risk of heart attack, for example, are related to high-cholesterol diets, a problem which is naturally avoided with a vegetarian lifestyle. A well-balanced vegetarian diet is also an effective, long-term solution to controlling excessive weight gain, which is in itself one of the high-risk factors for certain disorders, such as diabetes, gout, cholesterol, arteriosclerosis and high blood pressure.

In addition, a vegetarian diet is healthier in that we are not cumulatively absorbing as many potentially harmful additives as we might unknowingly do in a meat-rich diet, due to the pesticides, artificial growth hormones and high amounts of antibiotics that are commonly used in modern cattle feed, along with the chemical softeners, preservatives and colouring agents that are often added to the meat.

What is more, important food components, such as fibre and certain vitamins, are commonly found in particular plant foods, plus a lacto-vegetarian diet provides a healthy energy balance; while a meat-based diet is generally too rich in energy and a vegan diet tends to be on the lower end of the energy scale.

Increasing physical and mental efficiency

Yoga postures and breathing exercises provide countless benefits to all the body's systems and meditation builds up mental strength. However, bad eating habits can reduce the benefits you gain from yoga practice. By contrast, a well-balanced vegetarian diet is proven to greatly enhance and prolong the effects of yoga. Proper diet is an important pillar in the five points of yoga (see pages 10–11), which will allow you to face the physical and mental challenges of daily life more easily.

According to yoga, the subtle part of the food creates the energy for the thinking processes. This idea of 'food for thought' makes perfect sense in scientific terms: like all other cells of the body, the neurons in the brain need to absorb specific nutrition in order to function properly. Eating fresh plant food, which has absorbed maximum sunlight, is the best source for physical and mental strength.

Adapting to vegetarian ways

When changing to a vegetarian lifestyle, it is best to focus firstly on discovering the many healthy food items that are available, rather than forcing yourself to give up habitual parts of your present diet. In this way you avoid any psychological pressure and potential deficiencies from a sudden change. Discover and experiment with the staple vegetarian foods: whole grains such as wheat, brown rice, millet, barley, oats, quinoa and corn;

pulses such as lentils, chickpeas, mung beans, toor dhal, aduki beans and soya products; the many varieties of seasonal fruit and vegetables from your local organic market; various nuts; and also seeds, which can be consumed in a highly energetic sprouted form, such as alfalfa and sunflower seeds.

It may well take your body a while to adjust to the lower energy intake of a vegetarian diet. At first, this may lead to an excessive consumption of concentrated dairy products, such as heavy cheeses or a strong craving for sweets. While paying attention to the minimum quantity of both dairy products and sweets, it is important to try out as many new vegetarian combinations and recipes as possible. Variety will contribute to both a better supply of nutrients and greater enjoyment during meals.

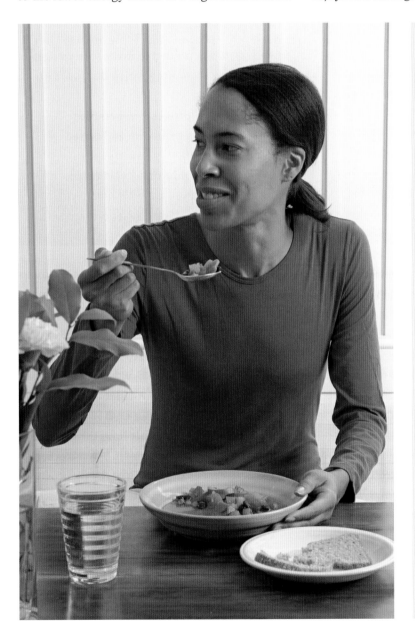

Essential ingredients

Many studies have proven that the consumption of a variety of plant foods as well as a small amount of dairy products supply all the basic nutrients in optimal amounts. However, in order to combine vegetarian foods in the proper proportions to promote a healthy life, you need to take on board some basic nutritional facts (see pages 132–133 for more information on how to obtain these nutrients).

• Carbohydrates and fats are the main energy suppliers, allowing all the body's organs and systems to perform their functions.

• Proteins, minerals and water are required for the continuous renewal of cells and tissues.

• Vitamins and minerals are needed to regulate body processes and are essential for the work of hormones and enzymes in the body.

YOGIC DIET

Besides the many nutritional aspects of this vegetarian diet, the following section focuses on how a well-balanced diet also relates to the benefits of yoga exercises.

Ideally, yoga should be practised either before breakfast or before dinner. A proper meal not long after the practice, however, can enhance and prolong the relaxing and energizing effects of the exercises.

The three *gunas*

According to yogic teachings, *prana* vibrates in three frequency ranges or qualities of nature called *gunas*:

Sattwa – purity, balance
Rajas – activity, passion
Tamas – inertia, sleep

These qualities can be observed in nature, in the body and in the mind. At any given time, there is a natural predominance of one of them. Yoga postures, breathing exercises and relaxation techniques activate the flow of these three forms of *prana*, progressively unblocking stagnation or excess of *tamas*, reducing the hyperactive tendencies of *rajas* and promoting the balancing effect of *sattwa*. Yoga develops our pure inner nature and diet plays a very important part in this process.

Food can also be classified according to these three categories. By introducing more *sattwic* elements into your meals, while avoiding *rajasic* and *tamasic* food items, you can actively enhance and prolong the balancing effect of your yoga practice, calm the mind and sharpen the intellect.

Sattwic foods

Sattwic foods help to increase vitality, energy, health and joy, and are conducive to the practice of yoga. They include: grains such as corn, barley, wheat, rice, oats, millet and quinoa; pulses, nuts and seeds; vegetables, especially leafy green ones, such as broccoli, spinach and chard, and seeded vegetables, such as cucumbers and squashes; fruit, both fresh and dried; natural sweeteners, such as honey, molasses, maple syrup; and dairy products in small quantities, such as milk, butter, light cheeses and yoghurt.

Rajasic foods

The over-stimulating effect of *rajasic* foods can create both physical and mental stress. Foods and drinks that fall into this category should therefore be consumed in moderation. They include: onions, garlic, radishes, coffee, tea and other stimulants (especially ones that contain the chemical taurine), refined (white) sugar, soft drinks, pungent spices, highly seasoned foods and anything that is excessively hot, bitter, salty or sour. As you continue your yoga practice, you will become more sensitive to these over-stimulating influences.

Tamasic foods

Tamasic foods are thought to make a person feel tired and inert. Meat, fish, eggs, alcoholic beverages and drugs are all *tamasic* in nature.

Stale, rotten, fermented, burnt, fried, reheated and canned food also have a *tamasic* effect, as does over-ripe and unripe fruit. Reducing and finally eliminating *tamasic* food items from your overall diet is an important step to improving your quality of life.

AYURVEDIC ADVICE

Although the human body comes in many shapes and sizes, every individual can be classified, to some extent, as belonging to one of three basic body types – ectomorph, mesomorph and endomorph. The ancient Indian health science of Ayurveda is a sister science of yoga and has developed a unique nutrition system based on the dietary needs of these three body types. As well as body type, your age, the type of work you do, the climate you live in and the current season all affect which foods are best for you and when to eat them.

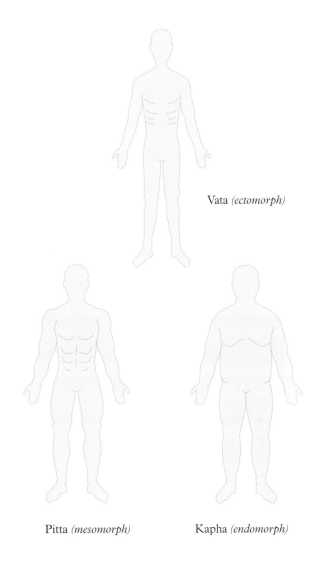

Vata *(ectomorph)*

Pitta *(mesomorph)*   Kapha *(endomorph)*

Vata or air type (ectomorph)

A *vata* constitution is typically of thin build and has delicate bone structure, limited muscular development, thin hair, dry skin and a low digestive fire, which means less secretion of gastric juices in the stomach and duodenum, so slower digestion. A *vata* diet should consist of up to five small meals evenly spread throughout the day. This body type requires mostly warm food, quite well-spiced and with a good quantity of easily digestible fats, for example, cold-pressed plant oils either added to the food while cooking or upon serving. Fats that are difficult to digest, including deep-fried foods or fat contained in frozen or microwaved food, should be avoided.

Pitta or fire type (mesomorph)

People with a typically *pitta* body are of medium height, weight and bone strength, with soft, warm skin, prematurely white or thinning hair, a strong digestive fire (good digestion) and a healthy appetite. Even though this body type can digest most food items well, an unbalanced diet will still have its long-term degenerative effects. A *pitta* diet should not include hot spices.

Kapha or water/earth type (endomorph)

A *kapha* person has a well-developed body, a large ribcage, well-defined muscles, a tendency to easily become overweight, strong, soft hair and slightly oily skin. While the appetite of a *kapha* person tends to be regular, the digestive function is slow, so food intake should be moderate. Well-spiced food and a good amount of raw food items are helpful for this body type.

GOOD DIGESTION

It is just as important to watch how well you are digesting, absorbing and eliminating food as it is to eat healthy food in the first place. This is all the more important in the rushed, pressurized lives that most of us lead today, where we so often only manage to eat 'on the move' or in a hurry between one job and the next. No matter how much 'good food' we feed ourselves, it will be of no use to us if our body is being placed under too much strain to actually process it.

Improving digestion

Digestion begins with chewing and mixing your food with saliva in your mouth. Practically speaking, it means that you should thoroughly chew (break down) and swallow each mouthful of food before even considering putting the next portion into your mouth. Your stomach then acts like a blender, mixing the food with its acidic digestive juices. If your stomach is too full, or the pieces of food in it are too big, it cannot blend the food easily.

Yoga advises to fill half of the stomach with solid food, a quarter with liquids and leave the remaining quarter empty. It takes 20 minutes for the stomach to be able to communicate a natural feeling of saturation. This means that if you eat a meal hastily, for example within ten minutes, your stomach will not feel full, even if it was a supposedly filling meal. Slow, relaxed eating is therefore necessary to allow your stomach to function properly.

The secretion of digestive juices is regulated by the autonomic (involuntary) nervous system. Stress activates sympathetic nerve impulses within this system that slow down digestion, whereas relaxation activates parasympathetic

nerve impulses which boost circulation in the digestive organs and enhance the peristaltic movement (the series of muscular contractions through the digestive tract that push the food from the oesophogus down to the anus). You should therefore avoid taking your meals under stress, especially if you have a naturally low digestive fire (see the information on body types on page 135). When you feel particularly worried or stressed, try to relax on your back in Corpse Pose for 5–10 minutes before a meal, whenever possible (see pages 28–29).

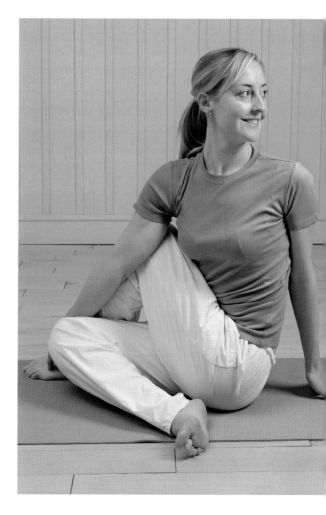

It is also important to ensure that your body is eliminating waste products at a healthy rate – the by-products of the process of digestion. If it is not doing this efficiently, such as in the case of constipation, it means that toxins can build up within your system, making you feel heavy, lethargic and, in some cases, even ill.

Regular exercise, more fibre in your diet, adequate water intake and eating a few soaked figs or prunes every morning are some of the common suggestions to improve elimination. Asanas such as the Plough (see pages 72–73), Forward Bend (see pages 76–77), the Bow (see pages 96–97), Half Spinal Twist (see pages 98–101) and the Peacock (see page 117) also help to activate the peristaltic movement, which should prevent any blockages.

Fasting

Fasting is a good, natural way to maintain optimal health and overcome many diseases. During a fast, the complete lack of new food intake gives your body time to process and eliminate what is already in there, so that it does not build up as 'toxic waste'.

A simple and safe form of fasting is a 24-hour fast. On the day of the fast, try to drink at least 2 litres (3½ pints) of mild herbal teas such as fennel, chamomile or linden, as well as plain mineral water. If you have a juicer, you can drink four large glasses of fresh carrot juice mixed with a few drops of olive oil throughout the day, as this makes the fast more pleasant. Taking an evening walk and relaxing with a hot-water bottle on your stomach will help you to sleep well.

No special precautions are needed to break this one-day fast the next day. However, chewing your food well and eating smaller meals than normal in the days that follow will prolong the sense of well-being and increased vitality you

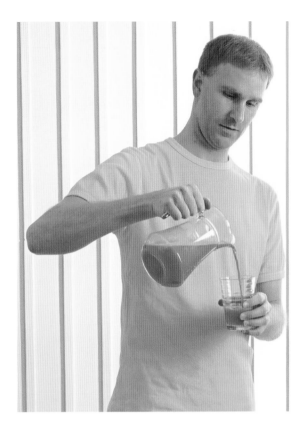

enjoy after the fast. The 24-hour fast can be done once every seven to ten days.

Longer fasting sessions require expert guidance, as the production of digestive juices stops and the peristaltic movement slows down, which means that enemas and special salts are required to maintain proper elimination. Such a fast would need to be broken gradually over at least half the time of the actual fasting period, supervised by an expert the whole time.

Fasting is a time-proven way to develop both your mental and spiritual faculties. It imposes a break on the mechanical habit of eating and develops willpower, which in turn improves concentration. The senses are naturally withdrawn from seeing, smelling and tasting food and *prana* is rejuvenated while fasting. All these factors will enhance your meditation practice (see pages 146–155).

YOGA CLEANSING EXERCISES

Regular intake of food is needed for absorption of life force, or *prana*. The body requires about a third of its *prana* to digest, absorb and eliminate it. When the process of elimination is impaired, the accumulated waste products have a toxic effect in the body and block the proper flow of vital energy.

Many internal organs are lined with mucous membranes, which constantly produce new mucus. This traps pollutants, humidifies the air in the respiratory tract, and in the digestive system it protects the organs from the strong acidity of the digestive juices and allows the food to move smoothly through the system. When people have an excessive amount of mucus accumulating in their organs, it creates a heavy feeling in the whole body.

Yoga cleansing exercises, known as *kriyas*, help the body to get rid of such excess mucus. They do this by increasing the blood circulation in many organs and therefore stimulating the elimination of toxins from many tissues.

Uddhiyana bandha

This *kriya* massages the digestive organs, increasing blood circulation to them and enhancing their performance. It is best to practise it in the morning on an empty stomach.

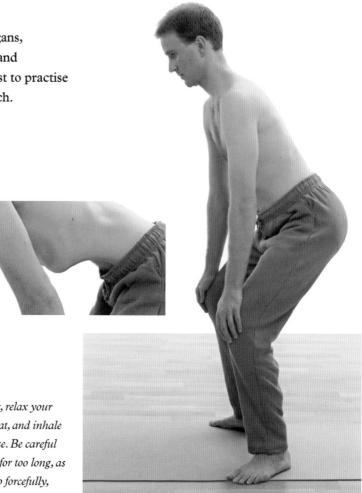

1 *Stand with your legs apart and your hands on your thighs close to your knees. Keeping your arms quite straight, bend your knees and bend forwards slightly. After a deep inhalation, forcibly exhale through both your nose and mouth, and hold your breath. Then progressively contract your abdomen until it is pulled in and up, applying maximum pressure to the internal organs.*

2 *After a few seconds, relax your abdomen and throat, and inhale slowly through your nose. Be careful not to hold your breath for too long, as you may then inhale too forcefully, which can hurt your throat and lungs.*

Jala neti

Most people brush their teeth, blow their noses and clear their throats every day. However, these techniques do not reach the back of the nasal cavity and the passage to the oral cavity, which are where many common colds begin. In the yogic exercise called *Jala neti* (nasal cleansing with water), warm salt water is made to flow from one nostril to the other and from the nose into the mouth in order to eliminate excess mucus.

A tool known as a *neti* pot is required for this exercise. These are available in most health food stores and online shops. Fill it with warm tap water and add sea salt until the water has a moderately salty taste. Besides having an antiseptic effect, the right amount of salt in the water will prevent any kind of burning sensation from occurring.

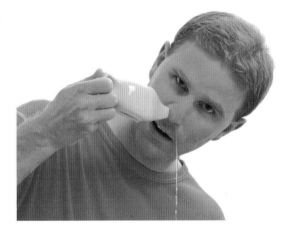

1 *Bend over the sink, put the opening of the* neti *pot against one nostril and breathe in and out freely through your mouth. Then bend your head to the side until the water flows out through the other nostril. After a few seconds, come back to standing position, blow your nose and then do the same on the other nostril. Be careful not to bend too much to the side, as this can cause water to enter from the oral cavity to the ears, causing discomfort.*

2 *Next, try to make the water flow from your nose into your mouth. Take a deep inhalation and hold your breath. Use one hand to put the opening of the* neti *pot against one nostril and your other hand to close the other nostril. Lift your head and start to make a gargling sound with a long exhalation. As the water flows from your nose into your throat, the gargling should push the water up into your mouth. When you have completed the exhalation, bend over and let the water flow from your nose and mouth into the sink. After a few seconds, return to a standing position, blow your nose and then, do the same on the other nostril. Be careful not to lift your head too much, as this may cause water to enter the frontal sinuses (the cavities between the nose and forehead), creating uncomfortable pressure.*

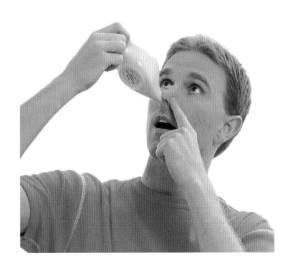

QUICK AND EASY MENUS

The following pages provide you with some delicious vegetarian recipes that will help you in your transition towards a healthier, more balanced and life. Options are given for breakfast, lunch and dinner, using many of the health-giving ingredients mentioned in the preceding pages.

Breakfast

Almond milk

This sustaining and soothing drink was developed by Swami Vishnu-devananda during the time that he was doing intensive *sadhana* (yogic practice) in the Himalayas. It is a rich source of easily digestible food for the rapid replenishment of energy. *Serves 1*

10 almonds, covered in water and soaked overnight
pinch of ground cardamom
pinch of pepper
250 ml (8 fl oz) warm milk, water or soya milk
1 teaspoon honey

1 Drain the almonds, keeping the soaking water, and remove the skins. Place the nuts in a food processor or blender with the soaking water, the cardamom and pepper. Blend at high speed for 5 minutes.

2 Combine the almond mixture with the warm milk, water or soya milk. Then stir in the honey and drink immediately.

Fruit toast

An interesting departure from the more traditional cinnamon toast, this recipe needs a little preparation, but is a wonderfully satisfying breakfast. Any seasonal fruit may be used. *Serves 1*

1 teaspoon butter or margarine
1 peach, nectarine or apple, or 2 apricots sliced
2 teaspoons sugar-free whole fruit apricot or peach jam
1 teaspoon lemon juice (optional)
1 slice light rye or sunflower seed bread, lightly toasted

1 Preheat the oven to 200°C/400°F/Gas mark 6. Melt the butter or margarine in a large, heavy-based saucepan or frying pan and sauté the fruit for 2–3 minutes, until it begins to soften. Turn off the heat and stir in the fruit jam and lemon juice, if using.

2 Place the toast on a baking sheet and spoon the fruit mixture on top of it. Bake in the oven for 5–10 minutes and serve immediately.

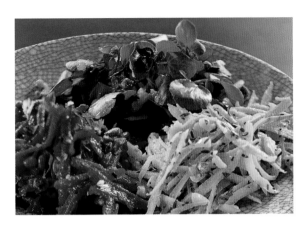

Lunch

Roasted tomato soup

Simple, wholesome foods like this soup help to maintain physical health and mental equilibrium. Roasting the tomatoes first creates more of an exotic flavour. *Serves 4–6*

450 g (1 lb) tomatoes
2 tablespoons oil
1 red pepper, cored, seeded and chopped
1 carrot, grated
2 sticks of celery, sliced
1 tablespoon chopped fresh oregano or ¾ teaspoon dried
1 tablespoon torn fresh basil or 1 teaspoon dried
750 ml (1¼ pints) hot water
1 teaspoon salt
¼ teaspoon pepper
basil and oregano leaves or 2 tablespoons chopped fresh parsley to garnish

1 Preheat the oven to 200°C/400°F/Gas mark 6 and roast the whole tomatoes, turning frequently until the skins fall away (about 15 minutes). Cool slightly, then peel and chop.

2 Heat the oil in a pan and sauté the pepper, carrot and celery over a medium heat for a few minutes. Add the oregano and basil, stir well and cook for a few more minutes.

3 Add the water and tomatoes, season with salt and pepper, half cover and simmer for about 20 minutes. Transfer to a food processor or blender and blend for a few seconds. Return the soup to the pan and reheat if necessary. Then serve garnished with fresh basil and oregano leaves or chopped parsley.

Tri-coloured salad

The colours and tastes of this healthy salad platter complement each other wonderfully. *Serves 4–6*

BEETROOT SALAD
4 raw beetroot, grated
100 g (4 oz) sunflower seeds, roasted
1 tablespoon chopped fresh thyme or tarragon
250 ml (8 fl oz) crème fraîche

WATERCRESS SALAD
100 g (4 oz) walnut pieces
1 bunch watercress, trimmed
1 green pepper, cored, seeded and sliced
juice of 1 grapefruit
125 ml (4 fl oz) olive oil
salt and pepper to taste

CARROT SALAD, INDIAN-STYLE
2 carrots, shredded
1 teaspoon salt (optional)
1 tablespoon raw unsalted peanuts
1 tablespoon oil
½ teaspoon cumin seeds
½ teaspoon black mustard seeds
1 teaspoon sesame seeds
pinch of ground coriander
¼ teaspoon cayenne pepper
1 teaspoon lemon or lime juice
2 tablespoons chopped fresh coriander

1 To make the beetroot salad, simply combine all the ingredients.

2 To make the watercress salad, heat a heavy frying pan and roast the walnuts over a high heat until browned. Leave to cool, then mix with the watercress and green pepper. In a separate bowl, combine the grapefruit juice, olive oil, salt and pepper and pour this over the watercress mixture.

3 To make the carrot salad, place the carrots in a bowl and stir in the salt. Roast the peanuts in a frying pan, stirring until they have turned a darker colour and are giving off a rich aroma. Allow the peanuts to cool and grind them coarsely. Heat the oil in a small pan and roast all the seeds until they 'pop'. Add the ground coriander and cayenne pepper to the seeds and cook for 1 minute, stirring constantly. Stir the mixture into the carrots, with the peanuts, lemon or lime juice and chopped coriander.

4 Arrange the salads on a large serving plate.

Dinner

Aubergine quinoa roast

The high-energy grain quinoa – from South America's Andes mountains – is given an international flavour in this vegetable-rich dish, and needs only a green salad to complement it. *Serves 4*

4 tablespoons sesame oil
350 g (12 oz) aubergine, cut into 8 thick slices
2 tablespoons tamari
50 ml (2 fl oz) lemon juice
125 ml (4 fl oz) water
1 teaspoon grated fresh root ginger
200 g (7 oz) quinoa, washed
1 large red pepper, cored, seeded and sliced
2 courgettes, coarsely grated
parsley sprigs, to garnish

1 Preheat the oven to 180°C/350°F/Gas mark 4. Heat the sesame oil in a frying pan and cook the aubergine slices until browned. Retain the oil and arrange the aubergine in a single layer in a baking dish. Combine the tamari, lemon juice, water and ginger and pour this over the aubergine slices. Bake in the oven for 10 minutes. Turn the slices over and cook for 10 minutes, until most of the liquid has been absorbed.

2 Place the quinoa in a large pan with double its volume of water. Bring to the boil, cover and simmer for 15 minutes, until tender. Drain if necessary. Add the red pepper and courgettes to the sesame oil remaining in the frying pan and sauté until soft. Add the quinoa, mix well and spoon over the aubergine. Press down well. Return to the oven and cook for 5–10 minutes. Serve hot, garnished with parsley sprigs.

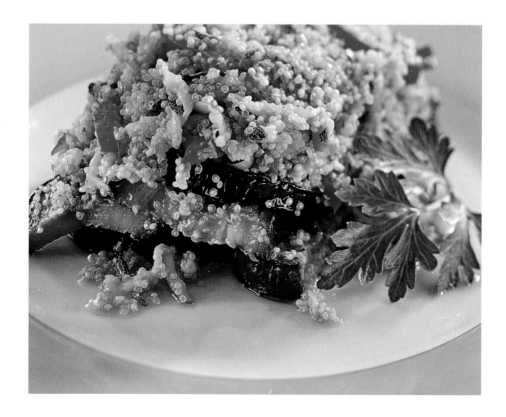

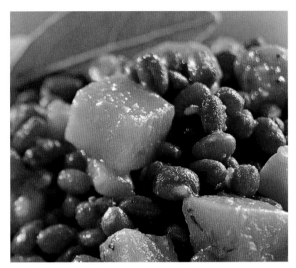
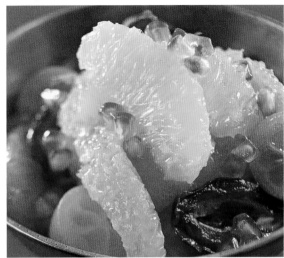

Aduki bean stew

Aduki beans are used extensively in Japanese cooking. This is a classic macrobiotic dish, best served on rice or millet. *Serves 4–6*

175 g (6 oz) aduki beans, soaked
2 bay leaves (optional)
900 ml (1½ pints) water
300 g (10 oz) acorn or butternut squash, peeled, seeded and cut into small cubes
1 carrot, cubed or sliced
½ teaspoon dried thyme
2–4 tablespoons miso

1 Drain the beans and place in a pan with the bay leaves and water. Cook over a medium heat for about 40 minutes, until almost tender, adding a little more water if necessary.

2 Add the squash, carrot and thyme. Continue to simmer for about 20 minutes, until everything is tender, stirring occasionally. The stew should have a slightly dry consistency. Remove the pan from the heat and stir in the miso. Serve at once.

Fragrant fruit salad

This delicious combination of fresh ingredients offers the perfect ending to a meal, without bringing your body out of balance in any way. If fresh figs or dates are unavailable, use dried, pre-soaked in cold water for 30 minutes. *Serves 4–6*

2 oranges
½ teaspoon orange flower water
1–2 tablespoons honey or date syrup (optional)
1 pink grapefruit
8 kumquats, halved, or 16 cherries
100 g (4 oz) fresh dates or figs, halved and cut lengthwise
pomegranate seeds

1 Squeeze the juice from one orange and combine it with the orange flower water and honey or date syrup, if using this, to make a syrup. Remove all skin and pith from the other orange and the grapefruit, dividing them into segments.

2 Arrange the orange and grapefruit over the other fruits in a bowl and pour the syrup over them. Sprinkle with pomegranate seeds and chill before serving.

CHAPTER 3

Meditation

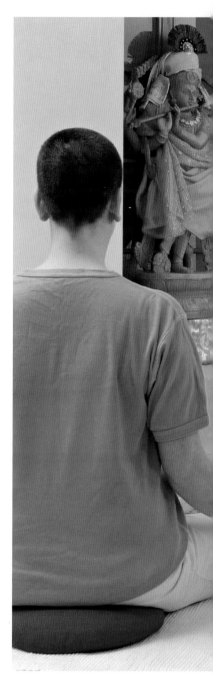

'In meditating regularly, the mind becomes clearer and clearer, and the motives become more and more pure. The subconscious releases hidden knowledge that allows understanding of the ways in which each binds himself in daily habits. The ego is slowly eradicated by concentration on a broader awareness of the universe and one's relation to it. Ultimately the superconscious, or intuitive forces, are released, leading to a life of wisdom and peace.'
Swami Vishnu-devananda

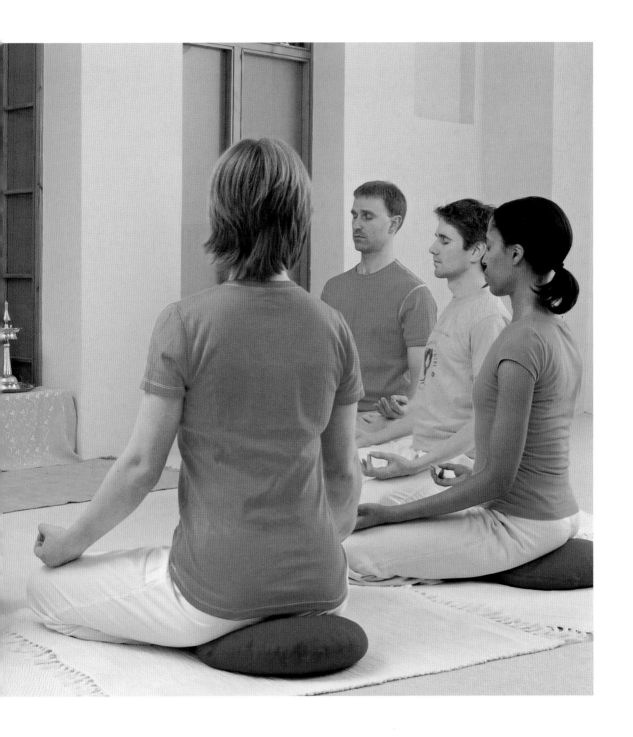

THE WORKINGS OF THE MIND

The mind is not a visible, tangible thing. According to yoga, it is made up of subtle energy, or *prana*, which is constantly influenced by our physical surroundings and by the people with whom we interact, as well as by the general atmosphere in which we live.

The ever-moving mind

When you are not aware of the constant fluctuation of your mind, the imagination runs free. This lack of conscious control over your own thoughts may initially seem pleasant. However, when more and more doubts crop up and superficial desires start to occupy your mind (often without you even realizing), life can become complicated. The luxury of today becomes the necessity of tomorrow, and the mind becomes anxious with thoughts, such as: 'What do other people think about me?', 'This person earns more than me, so must be happier than me', and 'That person is more talented than me, so must be better than me.' If we compare the mind to a lake, these thoughts are like waves that rise and fall on the surface, preventing us from seeing the calm waters that lie beneath – obscuring the lake's true nature, and therefore the true, peaceful nature of our soul. Yoga – and in particular meditation – aims to still such thoughts, impulses, emotions and moods so that we can move towards finding this peace.

Visualization, attention and concentration

The inherent capacities of visualization, attention and concentration are applied naturally in daily life to a certain extent. For example, a fashion designer first visualizes a new dress; then pays attention to a variety of steps related to the idea, such as the material, technical aspects of the production and how to sell it; and finally applies mental capacities such as memory, willpower, logic, enthusiasm and faith with firm concentration in order to realize the creation.

According to yogic teachings, the satisfaction experienced both during the process and at the successful completion of the new design is actually not related to the external achievement. Happiness is, instead, the result of the concentrated state of mind in itself, just as the bottom of a lake becomes visible when the waves on the surface subside. In other words, quality of experience does not lie in external objects, but within ourselves (the subjects).

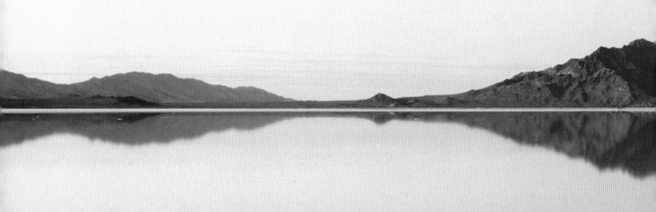

Calming the mind

Meditation practice allows you to consciously develop the capacities of visualization, attention and concentration. It is highly rewarding to become more aware of the inner workings of your own mind and to learn how to tune into the subtle experience of peace within. What is more, the mind becomes more flexible and therefore more able to adapt to all sorts of situations in daily life with greater ease.

Meditation requires an openness to a new perspective regarding body and mind: an awareness that the thinker is different from the thought. Your mind is as much your 'property' and outside of yourself as the limbs of your body, the clothes you wear or the building you live in. During meditation, each emotion, mood and sentiment that arises in the mind can be:

• firstly, separated – which category of thought is occurring?

• secondly, gently dissected – what is really hidden under the thought?

• and thirdly, analyzed – what is the motive of this thought and what will be its effect?

These steps allow each aspect of the mind to settle down and become calm.

Inner silence – inner strength

The body regenerates itself during the silence of sleep. When we dream, the mind relives impressions of the waking state and also satisfies desires that have not been gratified during the waking state. What is called 'good sleep' is actually the deep sleep in which oneness with the Self, or the subject, is experienced. And for general well-being, we need to experience this silent regeneration every day.

While dream and deep sleep are involuntary functions, meditation is a *conscious* way of attaining this peace and regeneration. It gives complete rest to the nervous system, promotes clarity of mind and connects us to our inner spiritual strength. Just as any amount of zeros has no value unless a one is put in front of it, so true well-being depends on the connection to the inner Self, or the subject.

Meditation gives a refreshing and exhilarating spiritual bath to body, mind and spirit. It is the key to the most priceless treasure we can own – intuitive wisdom. The peace of meditation gives deeper purpose to life and offers a means of simplifying and clarifying many complicated situations in life.

POSITIVE THINKING

In order to maintain inner strength in daily life, you need to develop a positive thought background and an ideal of how to live. These depend on a clear sense of discrimination regarding the effects of different types of thinking. It is essential to realize the ruinous consequences of negative thoughts.

Regular practice of yoga postures, good breathing techniques and relaxation exercises (see Chapter 1), as well as of meditation sessions (see pages 152–155), will stimulate your inner capacity to find and maintain a suitable 'ideal'. Positive thinking and meditation are, after all, one of the five basic principles of yoga (see pages 10–11). Just as muscle strength is developed by physical exercise, so psychic strength can be developed by mental exercise.

Cultivating thought power

Positive qualities such as truthfulness and earnestness are the best sources of mental strength to work towards. Concentration is also an invaluable quality to cultivate: the more concentration that can be developed in daily life, the more power can be brought to bear on one point. The development of willpower is also important. Much time and energy is wasted in the hankering for little daily comforts, so even by conquering one single habitual desire, you will notice an increase in willpower.

An unruffled state of mind, cheerfulness, inner strength, success in all undertakings, power to influence people, a magnetic and dynamic personality, sparkling eyes, a steady gaze, a powerful voice, an unyielding nature and fearlessness are just some of the signs which indicate your inner strength is growing.

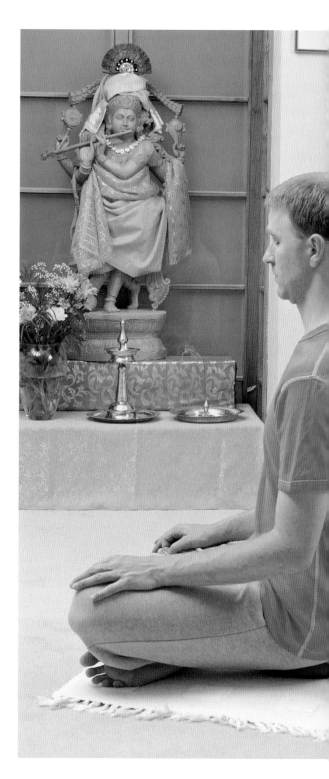

Physical and mental health

A healthy body creates a healthy mind. And in turn, healthy thoughts and emotions help to maintain a healthy body, while negative ones breed illness. Fits of hot temper, intense passion, bitter jealousy and corroding anxiety, for example, do serious damage to our brain cells, throw toxic chemicals into our blood and generally shock the system, draining away vitality and inducing premature old age. Cheerfulness and laughter, on the other hand, are tonics for the body. They boost the circulation, release 'happiness hormones' called endorphins and can counteract many imaginary ills. Even when you do have a certain health problem, thinking about it constantly will only serve to intensify it. Once appropriate medical diagnosis and treatment have been given, the best remedy is to practise positive thinking. As you think, so you become.

A powerful tool to help you with this are self-affirmations – positive statements about yourself, which you repeat when necessary in order to get you into a more positive frame of mind. Try, for example: 'I am healthy in body and mind. I am a storehouse of health, strength, vigour and vitality. I am the diseaseless Self or Soul. I am becoming better and better, day by day, in every way.' However, you could make up your own self-affirmations if you prefer.

Breaking the chains of negativity

At times, you may feel like a helpless victim of negative emotional impulses such as fear, anger, jealousy or impatience. You may find yourself justifying your negative emotional reactions as if they are the result of your environment, for example: 'I was afraid, because of the angry way she looked at me' or 'I got annoyed because of his rude behaviour'. This negative inner dialogue can continue for hours and sometimes days – like

Mutual attraction of thoughts

Like attracts like. People with similar thoughts tend to be attracted to each other. You could travel for months from country to country in search of something new. But inadvertently, you are always likely to attract to yourself only what corresponds to your own dominant quality of thought. It is therefore entirely in your own hands who you attract, as it is you, and you alone, who can determine the thoughts you entertain. The stillness of meditation can help you to create new, more positive, thought patterns.

a chain, its effect is to bind you to apparently unavoidable circumstances.

However, when you lift your thought energy to a higher wavelength via positive thinking, no negative external impact can bind you. You will then be able to express higher emotions, such as courage, love and contentment, whatever the external circumstances – without an inner dialogue such as 'Oh, how wonderfully patient I was with this irritated person.' Positive thinking is not a strategy; it is simply a natural expression of inner spiritual strength, which opens the way to true freedom of thought.

A negative thought is thrice cursed: it creates damage to the mind and body of the thinker, it creates negativity in the person to whom it is directed and it connects the thinker to the collective thought patterns of a similar nature.

A positive thought is thrice blessed: it creates vibrant mental and physical health in the thinker, it promotes well-being in others and it attracts positive reactions from the collective mass of positive thought energy.

FROM THOUGHT TO DESTINY

The law of cause and effect, or action and reaction, is prevalent on all physical and mental levels. Through this law, thoughts, actions and habits are intricately interwoven and create what most people consider destiny or fate. The regular practice of meditation can help you to become more aware of, clarify and even, potentially, change your thought processes – thus eventually clarifying and changing your destiny:

'You sow a thought and you reap an action'

In human law, not only is the action taken into account, but also the motive or 'thought' behind it. For example, there is a more severe punishment for a premeditated crime than for an impulsive one. The effect of any action therefore depends on the clarity and strength of the thought behind the action. Meditation is extremely helpful in promoting the development of pure, positive and peaceful thoughts within, unaffected by the surrounding external chaos.

'You sow an action and you reap a habit'

Most daily actions are habitual. Activities such as driving a car, climbing up stairs and eating do not need to be reprogrammed consciously each time. While this is very useful from a practical point of view, certain 'bad habits' can creep in and lower our life quality. For example, all types of addictions, whether to tobacco, alcohol, sugar or television, are based on the power of habit. Yoga recommends a gradual control of such negative habits. When you offer the mind new ways to relax, to recharge and to focus – such as through meditation – previous habits naturally fade out.

'You sow a habit and reap a character'

Although a lot of a person's character may be inborn and depend on their childhood education, yogic teachings propose an ongoing process of self-education. This means that when a negative character trait expresses itself causing trouble of some kind, you are encouraged to try to identify the habitual action – and therefore the thought – through which the trait expresses itself. The habitual but unconscious use of certain words is one example of a negative action that can lead to a negative character, preventing the mind from developing higher thinking. Keeping a diary in which you note down your thoughts and feelings in carefully chosen words can help to clear the mist of habitual language.

'You sow a character and reap a destiny'

Have you ever wondered why negative events sometimes only seem to occur in your life and not in the lives of people around you? The more you understand the nature of thought, action, habit and character, the more you will move away from such a negative thoughts – in which you abdicate all responsibility for your own life – and accept that you are master of your own destiny and architect of your own future. Positive thought and action in the present will gradually override all negative effects of past action.

ANCIENT WISDOM IN MODERN LIFE

According to yoga philosophy there are four aims in human existence. These are righteousness (*dharma*), economic independence (*artha*), emotional satisfaction (*kama*) and spiritual realization (*moksha*). Meditation provides the main pathway to *moshka*, as long as the other yogic principles are also put into practice (see pages 10–11).

Dharma is a law operating in the universe by which the body, mind and everything else is kept in a state of harmony and integration. Respecting *dharma*, or moral value, means that you see the individual Self as part of a global network that provides harmony for every individual being.

The material needs of the body, known as *artha*, are also very important. Nobody can ignore these basic requirements, such as protection against heat and cold; the need for food and liquid, sun and rain, and so on.

Then, there are the aesthetic longings of the human personality, known as *kama*. Humans will not be made happy merely by eating, drinking, putting on clothes and having a house in which to live. The aesthetic longings include the expression of the five senses and the satisfaction of desires. While it is not good to over-indulge these longings, people who try to ignore them completely may be subject to intense anger or continuous irritation. Yoga recommends moderation in everything.

Finally, there is aspiration for *moshka*, or spiritual fulfillment. These eternal values should be given careful consideration, as they influence everything else in life. Just as you need the unconscious satisfaction of deep sleep, there is an inner urge to consciously experience inner peace.

These four aims in human existence should be considered carefully. When doing so, you will quickly become aware of imbalances in your daily life and where changes should be made. Otherwise, much of your yoga practice will be wasted. It will be just like trying to fill a pot that is leaking.

Yoga offers a variety of spiritual practices that promote movement towards fulfilment. The meditation practices on the following pages are the ideal way to start your journey on the path to deeper levels of consciousness and inner peace.

PHYSICAL MEDITATION

Rather then being just an exercise of the mind, meditation begins with specific ways to sit, to adjust the breath and to direct the senses. Follow the guidelines below to create the best conditions in both the nervous system and general metabolism for the mind to concentrate. Bear in mind, however, that meditation can only be properly practised once you have completed at least Classes 1 and 2 (see pages 26–83).

Just as a cup needs to be held steady for the liquid in it to become still, so too does the body need to sit in a firm, relaxed position in order for the mind to become calm. The meditative pose that follows requires a fine-tuning of

strength, flexibility, relaxation and balance. The practice of the basic asanas of the yoga session (see Chapter 1, pages 22–127) will help you to attain these qualities.

The triangular alignment of the cross-legged position – with the head and knees making up the three points of the triangle – provides a stable pose, and the straight, relaxed spine position eliminates stress from the nervous system.

If your lower back becomes tired, your legs feel tense or any pressure accumulates in your knees, try sitting on a firm pillow or folded blanket – just high enough to make you more comfortable in the pose.

The meditative pose

Sit cross-legged in a quiet, well-ventilated place, preferably facing the East (the energy of the rising sun) or the North (the magnetic currents). Make sure that your weight is on your sitting bones, and that your back, neck and head are aligned. Place your hands either on your knees, with both hands in the chin mudra position (see page 86), or loosely held together in your lap (see inset picture). Initially, sit like this for about five minutes, but progressively build up to about 30 minutes.

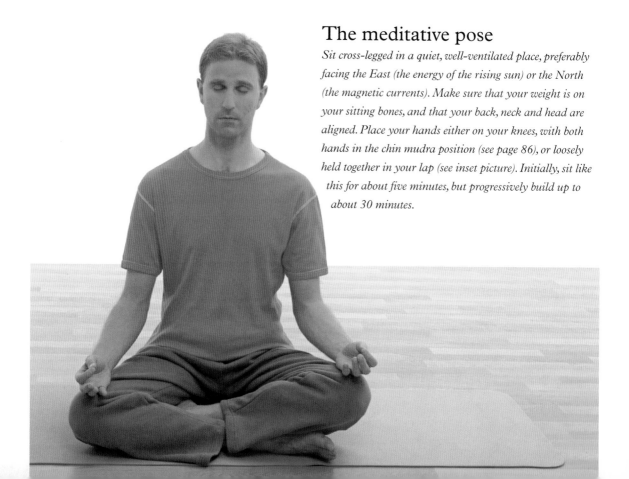

The meditative breath

The breath is an integral part of meditation: deep, steady breathing ensures a sufficient oxygen supply to the brain, promoting a state of concentrated relaxation and allowing your *prana*, or vital energy, to flow in a balanced way.

1 *Sitting cross-legged in the meditative pose, with your eyes closed, take a few Complete Yogic Breaths (see pages 60–63) to bring more oxygen to your brain. The active movement of all your respiratory muscles from your abdomen up to your chest will naturally align your spine.*

2 *Then practise Abdominal Breathing (see pages 38–41). Breathing both in and out through your nose, inhale for about 3 seconds and exhale for the same amount of time. Consciously send a message to all your muscles from your feet up to your head, telling them to relax – a process known as autosuggestion (see Step 10, page 55).*

3 *Now try to make the airflow in your nostrils as slow and smooth as possible. To start with, you may notice ups and downs in the air pressure, but as the coordination of your abdominal muscles and diaphragm improves, the airflow will become even. This is called* kevala kumbhaka *in Sanskrit. Practise for just 5 minutes at first and work up to 30 minutes.*

The meditative focus

The best time to practise this is after the Final Relaxation of the yoga session (see pages 54–57). Otherwise, any quiet moment in the morning or evening is good, but always spend a few minutes in the meditative pose, practising correct breathing, before you start to practise the focus.

Sitting cross-legged and breathing rhythmically, find your natural point of focus – either your third eye (the space between your eyebrows) or heart chakra (in the middle of your chest at the level of your heart). You can alternate between the focal points from one session to the next until you know which one works best for you, but once you find this, it is best not to change it. Make sure you keep your eyes completely relaxed throughout. As you breathe in and out, imagine that the airflow is actually moving through your point of focus. You are likely to lose your focus many times, but do not worry about this; training yourself to gently return to it is the whole point. Continue this process for 5 minutes at first and build up to 30 minutes over time.

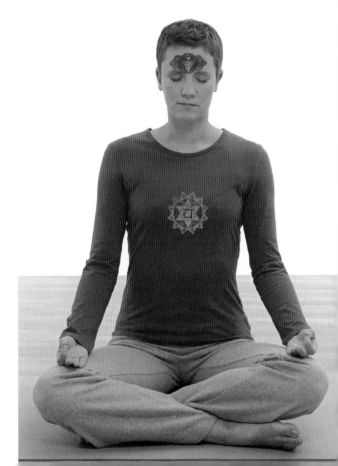

MEDITATION TECHNIQUES

Once you feel comfortable with physical meditation (see pages 152–153), you can start to add a specific object of meditation. Choose from the range of techniques that follow, according to your taste. All the exercises share the same purpose: to calm the mind and help you to experience inner peace, which is your real nature, just as the bottom of the lake is to water. Therefore simply practise whichever one works best for you, repeatedly over a prolonged period.

Tratak: Steady Gazing

This exercise may cause tears to flow but these will cleanse the eyes – acting as a *kriya*. The use of both actual sight and visualization make the meditation all the more powerful.

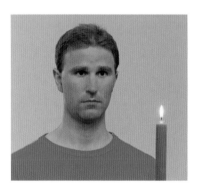

Sit cross-legged and place a lit candle at eye level in front of you. Breathe slowly and rhythmically, and gaze steadily for 1 minute at the brightest part of the flame, without blinking. Then close your eyes for 1 minute and visualize the image of the flame in the space between your eyebrows. Practise tratak *for up to 10 minutes, alternating 1-minute periods with your eyes open and closed.*

Nature Meditation

This meditative visualization draws on nature for inspiration. It is important, however, to exclude any emotional associations that you have with the natural object upon which you decide to focus.

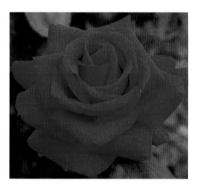

After several minutes of physical meditation, start to visualize an uplifting item from nature, such as a rose, in your chosen point of focus. Think of its colour and form, and of its various parts, such as the petals and the stalk. Visualize various kinds and colours of roses; bring to mind various preparations, such as rose water and rose perfume; and visualize roses in different ways – such as a bouquet, a garland or in a garden.

Mantra Meditation

The most direct concentration practice in yoga is mantra meditation or *japa* – repeating a sacred syllable or combination of syllables either internally or out loud. Normally, a word is considered only in relation to its meaning. For example, the word 'apple' makes sense only in connection with the mental image of an apple as something to be eaten. In a mantra, however, the vibrational set-up of the sound is such that it does not evoke a separate image or meaning.

In the beginning, it is best to meditate on the mantra OM, which is considered to be the universal sound of creation (see also page 30).

1 *Repeat OM out loud for up to 5 minutes at a comfortable pitch. Observe how various parts of your body resonate with the chanting sound. Then hold the vibration of M for as long as your exhalation naturally lasts.*

2 *Continue repeating OM silently for up to a further 10 minutes, synchronizing the sound with the point of focus and the breath: inhale OM and exhale OM.*

Abstract Meditation

Adding any of the following universal affirmations to an OM meditation will help you to develop a positive and expanded state of consciousness. It is important to be firmly connected with the practice of physical meditation (see pages 152–153) before doing this abstract meditation to prevent the mind from easily wandering away.

Sit cross-legged, breathe deeply and rhythmically, and alternate the internal repetition of OM with the internal repetition of the affirmation you choose. Do this for just 5 minutes at the start, but work up, over time, to do it for 30 minutes.

I am the All	*OM OM OM...*
I am the Immortal Self	*OM OM OM...*
I am the Light of Lights	*OM OM OM...*
I am the Sun of Suns	*OM OM OM...*
All Purity I am	*OM OM OM...*
All Bliss I am	*OM OM OM...*
Pure Consciousness	*OM OM OM...*

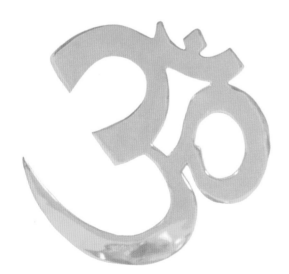

INDEX

SIVANANDA YOGA VEDANTA CENTRES

ASHRAMS

Sivananda Yoga Retreat House
Bichlach 40
A-6370 Reith bei Kitzbuhel
AUSTRIA
Tel: +43 5356 67 404
tyrol@sivananda.net

Sivananda Ashram Yoga Retreat
P.O. Box N7550
Paradise Island, Nassau
BAHAMAS
Tel: +1 242 363 2902
Nassau@sivananda.org

Sivananda Ashram Yoga Camp
673, 8th Avenue
Val Morin
Quebec J0T 2R0
CANADA
Tel: +1 819 322 3226
HQ@sivananda.org

Chateau du Yoga Sivananda
26 Impasse du Bignon
45170 Neuville aux Bois
FRANCE
Tel: +33 2 38 91 88 82
orleans@sivananda.net

Sivananda Yoga Vedanta
Dhanwantari Ashram
P.O.Neyyar Dam
Thiruvananthapuram Dt.
Kerala, 695 572
INDIA
Tel: +91 471 2273 093
YogaIndia@sivananda.org

Sivananda Yoga Vedanta
Meenakshi Ashram
Kalloothu, Saramthangi Village
Vellayampatti P.O., Palamedu (via)
Vadippatti Taluk, Madurai Dist.
625 503 Tamil Nadu
INDIA
Tel: +91 452 209 0662
madurai@sivananda.org

Sivananda Kutir
P.O. Netala, Uttara Kashi Dt
(near Siror Bridge)
Uttaranchal, Himalayas, 249 193
INDIA
Tel: +91 1374 222624
Tel: +91 1374 236296
himalayas@sivananda.org

Sivananda Ashram Yoga Farm
14651 Ballantree Lane, Comp. 8
Grass Valley, CA 95949
USA
Tel: +1 530 272 9322
Tel: 1-800-469-9642
YogaFarm@sivananda.org

Sivananda Ashram Yoga Ranch
P.O. Box 195, Budd Road
Woodbourne, NY 12788
USA
Tel: +1 845 436 6492
YogaRanch@sivananda.org

CENTRES

Centro Internacional de Yoga
Sivananda
Julian Alvarez 2201
CP 1425 Buenos Aires
ARGENTINA
Tel: +54 11 4827 9269
Tel: +54 11 4827 9566
BuenosAires@sivananda.org

Sivananda Yoga Vedanta Zentrum
Prinz-Eugenstrasse 18
A-1040 Vienna
AUSTRIA
Tel: +43 1 586 3453
Vienna@sivananda.net

Sivananda Yoga Vedanta Centre
5178 St Lawrence Blvd
Montreal, Quebec H2T 1R8,
CANADA
Tel: +1 514 279 3545
Montreal@sivananda.org

Sivananda Yoga Vedanta Centre
77 Harbord Street
Toronto, Ontario M5S 1G4,
CANADA
Tel: +1 416 966 9642
Toronto@sivananda.org

Centre Sivananda de Yoga Vedanta
123 Boulevard de Sebastopol
F-75002 Paris
FRANCE
Tel: +33 1 40 26 77 49
Tel: +33 1 42 33 51 97
Paris@sivananda.net

Sivananda Yoga Vedanta Zentrum
Steinheilstrasse 1
D-80333 Munich
GERMANY
Tel: +49 89 52 44 76
Munich@sivananda.net

Sivananda Yoga Vedanta Zentrum
Schmiljanstrasse 24
D-12161 Berlin
GERMANY
Tel: +49 30 85 99 97 98
Berlin@sivananda.net

Sivananda Yoga Vedanta Zentrum
(affiliated)
Kleiner Kielort 8
20144 Hamburg
GERMANY
Tel: +49 40 41 42 45 46
post@artyoga.de

Sivananda Yoga Vedanta
Nataraja Centre
A-41 Kailash Colony
New Delhi 110 048
INDIA
Tel: +91 11 2648 0869
Tel: +91 11 2645 3962
Delhi@sivananda.org

Sivananda Yoga Vedanta Centre
House No.18, TC 36/1238
Subhash Nagar
Vallakkadavu PO, Perunthanni,
Trivandrum,
695 008, Kerala
INDIA
Tel: +91 471 245 1398
Tel: +91 471 245 0942
Trivandrum@sivananda.org

Sivananda Yoga Vedanta Centre
3/655 (Plot No. 131) Kaveri Nagar
Kuppam Road
Kottivakkam, Chennai (Madras)
600 041
INDIA
Tel: +91 44 2451 1626
Tel: +91 44 2451 2546
e-mail: Madras@sivananda.org

Sivananda Yoga Vedanta Centre
Plot # 23, Dr Sathar Road
Anna Nagar, Madurai 625 025
Tamil Nadu
INDIA
Tel: +91 452 252 1170
maduraicentre@sivananda.org

Sivananda Yoga Vedanta Centre
6 Lateris St., Tel Aviv 64166,
ISRAEL
Tel: +972 3 691 6793
TelAviv@sivananda.org

Centro Yoga Vedanta Sivananda
Via Oreste Tommasini, 7
00162 Roma
ITALY
tel: + 39 06 45 49 65 28
rome@sivananda.org

Centro de Yoga Sivananda Vedanta
Calle Eraso 4, E-28028 Madrid
SPAIN
Tel: +34 91 361 5150
Madrid@sivananda.net

Centre Sivananda de Yoga Vedanta
1 Rue des Minoteries
CH-1205 Geneva,
SWITZERLAND
Tel: +41 22 328 03 28
Geneva@sivananda.net

Asociacion de Yoga Sivananda
Acevedo Diaz 1523
11200 Montevideo
URUGUAY
Tel: +598 2 401 09 29
Tel: +598 2 401 66 85
Montevideo@sivananda.org

Sivananda Yoga Vedanta Centre
51 Felsham Road
London SW15 1AZ
UNITED KINGDOM
Tel: +44 20 8780 0160
London@sivananda.net

Sivananda Yoga Vedanta Center
1246 Bryn Mawr
Chicago, IL 60660
USA
Tel: +1 773 878 7771
Chicago@sivananda.org

Sivananda Yoga Vedanta Centre
243 West 24th Street
New York, NY 10011
USA
Tel: +1 212 255 4560
NewYork@sivananda.org

Sivananda Yoga Vedanta Center
1200 Arguello Blvd
San Francisco, CA 94122
USA
Tel: +1 415 681 2731
SanFrancisco@sivananda.org

Sivananda Yoga Vedanta Center
13325 Beach Avenue
Marina del Rey, CA 90292
USA
Tel: +1 310 822 9642
LosAngeles@sivananda.org

ACKNOWLEDGEMENTS

The Sivananda Yoga Vedanta Centre would like to thank
Swami Sivadasananda, Yoga Acharya, for writing the
book and Swami Durgananda, Yoga Acharya, for
inspiring ideas and advice.

We would also like to thank the photographic models:
Swami Anantananda, Saraswati, Narayani, Bheema,
Chandra, Jyothi, Sarada Devi and Yamuna.

**Special photography © Octopus Publishing Group
Limited**/Mike Good.

Other photography: DigitalVision 154 right.
ImageSource 150–151. **Octopus Publishing Group
Limited** 8, 9, 20–21, 146–147, 155;
/Adrian Swift 141, 142, 143 right.

Executive Editor **Jo Godfreywood**
Managing Editor **Clare Churly**
Executive Art Editor **Leigh Jones**
Designer **Lucy Guenot**
Picture Librarian **Sophie Delpech**
Production Controller **Simone Nauerth**